Praise for
EMBRACE THE SUCK

"Resilience is key to overcoming all obstacles in life, of which there are many! *Embrace the Suck* masterfully guides the reader through measurable ways to optimize their personal fortitude and become their best self."

—Mark Owen, #1 *New York Times* best-selling
author of *No Easy Day* and *No Hero*

"The one constant that connects us all is that every single one of us is going to get knocked down in life. What defines us and our character is not just what we do next, but how we do it. Brent Gleeson recommends you embrace the suck and get after it. I agree. It's time to execute!"

—Jack Carr, *New York Times* best-selling
author of *Savage Son*

"This riveting step-by-step manual boils it down to the one founding principle we are taught in the SEAL Teams: you have to learn to 'embrace the suck.' I highly recommend this book to anyone looking to level up with a proven process to overcome the adversity we all face in life and business!"

—Jason Redman, US Navy SEAL (Retired),
New York Times best-selling author of *The Trident*
and *Overcome*

"Tough times don't last, but tough people do. Whether in business or in life, adversity is often viewed as the enemy. Mindset, however, is the antidote and solution. *Embrace the Suck* is a no-nonsense field manual that will empower anyone to turn adversity into an advantage so that you can overcome any setback and dominate life. Brent Gleeson delivers the goods through his real-world, in-the-trenches experience as a Navy SEAL warrior and leadership expert."

—Bedros Keuilian, best-selling author of *Man Up* and founder of Fit Body Boot Camp

"No matter how you define success, the path to achieving it will require determination and resilience in the darkest of moments. In this no-nonsense self-help guide, you'll learn that in order to fulfill your goals, you have to be willing to embrace the suck."

—Todd Hymel, CEO, Volcom

"A book like this deserves its own category. *Embrace the Suck* is a book about resilience, personal development, and self-mastery. Each chapter is full of engaging stories of Navy SEAL missions complemented with real-life application for readers. This book screams, *Take action with your life*. Indeed a work of art that I won't soon forget."

—Alex Sanfilippo

EMBRACE
THE
SUCK

THE NAVY SEAL WAY
TO AN EXTRAORDINARY LIFE

BRENT GLEESON

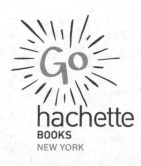

hachette
BOOKS
NEW YORK

Hachette Go, an imprint of Hachette Books
Hachette Book Group
1290 Avenue of the Americas
New York, NY 10104
HachetteGo.com
Facebook.com/HachetteGo
Instagram.com/HachetteGo

First Paperback Edition: December 2021

Hachette Books is a division of Hachette Book Group, Inc.

The Hachette Go and Hachette Books names and logos are trademarks of Hachette Book Group, Inc.

The publisher is not responsible for websites (or their content) that are not owned by the publisher.

Print book interior design by Jeff Williams.

Library of Congress Cataloging-in-Publication Data

Names: Gleeson, Brent, author.
Title: Embrace the suck : the Navy SEAL way to an extraordinary life / Brent Gleeson.
Description: First edition. | New York : Hachette Go, [2020] | Includes bibliographical references.
Identifiers: LCCN 2020014395 | ISBN 9780306846335 (hardcover) | ISBN 9780306846328 (ebook)
Subjects: LCSH: Resilience (Personality trait) | Success.
Classification: LCC BF698.35.R47 G54 2020 | DDC 158—dc23
LC record available at https://lccn.loc.gov/2020014395

ISBNs: 9780306846335 (hardcover), 9780306846342 (paperback), 9780306846328 (ebook)

Printed in the United States of America

LSC-C

Printing 3, 2023

CONTENTS

PART 3 TAKE ACTION: EXECUTE, EXECUTE, EXECUTE

FOREWORD

by David Goggins

*The pain that you are willing to endure is
measured by how bad you want it.*

—DAVID GOGGINS

Our minds are the most powerful weapon we have at our disposal. But often, our greatest tools can be exactly what stands in the way of overcoming adversity and achieving extraordinary accomplishments. If you can't learn to control your mind, you'll forever be a slave to its evil limitations.

I met Brent in late 2000 at the Naval Special Warfare Center in Coronado, California, when we joined Basic Underwater Demolition/SEAL class 235. I'd already been in SEAL training at the command for ten months, having endured two Hell Weeks and multiple injuries, but my journey in developing resilience and mental toughness was only just beginning.

I grew up in a physically and emotionally abusive household and battled learning disabilities, obesity, and racism every day. That environment fueled depression and a mindset consumed by fear and a deep need for acceptance of any kind. I was constantly trudging through the muck so to speak, with no end to the suffering in sight. One day, I realized that I could make the choice to rise from the ashes and take control of my life. In 1994, I joined the United States Air Force and served for five years as a tactical air controller. I found happiness and fulfillment in service to our great nation. Giving to a cause greater than myself filled a void I had struggled with for years. But after leaving the Air Force, depression pulled me back into its lonely lair. Down there in the darkness, what I lost in myself I regained in weight. And at 297 pounds, I became consumed by the fear of permanency; that was simply who I was going to be. At the time, I accepted it. Then one day, I looked in the mirror and said, "Fuck this." I decided to stop wallowing in misery, get off my ass, and start training. To take back control. Through extreme discipline and resolve, I lost 106 pounds in a very short period of time. In 2000, I joined the Navy with the goal of becoming a Navy SEAL.

I knew I'd have to dive headfirst into hell and battle the devil—even become the devil—to achieve this goal. I immersed myself in this new normal. I transformed my mind to embrace the pain, to enjoy it. I developed the mental calluses necessary to go to war with myself each day. Brent used to joke that I was possibly the only person in the history of the SEAL training program who relished the torture, that this battlefield had become my home. We completed what was my third Hell Week in March 2001. Eight months later, after completing SEAL Qualification

Training, Brent and I earned our Tridents and joined SEAL Team Five.

But it wasn't enough. I had become too comfortable in this new heightened state of performance. I needed to recertify myself as a savage and take my journey to the next level. As part of a cross-service training program after my first deployment, I opted to attend Army Ranger School. In 2004, I graduated from the program with the distinction of enlisted Top Honor Man and returned to Team Five. Soon after returning from Ranger School, I began my career as an elite ultramarathon athlete while on active duty as a SEAL.

I've been on a journey of self-discovery and comfort zone crushing ever since. Over the years, I've used my pain and suffering as fuel to drive me forward. I've become an accomplished endurance athlete, completing more than 60 ultramarathons, triathlons, and ultratriathlons, setting new course records and regularly placing in the top five. I once held the Guinness World Record for pull-ups, completing 4,030 in seventeen hours.

But all of the awards, medals, accolades, and magazine articles mean nothing to me. That's not why I do what I do. Sure, I have raised significant funds and awareness for the Special Operations Warrior Foundation, but I don't need the recognition. I'm not trying to be number one in the world at anything. It's not about how many races I run or how many miles I've traveled on broken feet. There's no scoreboard. Rather, it's about achieving my personal best and pushing well beyond my comfort zone every chance I get. For me, physical and mental suffering are a journey of introspection; no other experience makes me feel more clear, focused, and alive.

We all have the ability to master our minds. But our brains are wired with defense mechanisms for avoiding pain and hardship, for staying well within the confines of our comfort zone. Our minds have a tendency to force us into a sheltered existence. I call this the "forty percent rule." When our brains start sending signals that we can go no further, endure no more, to retreat to the blissful embrace of denial and mediocrity, we've only achieved forty percent of our mental and physical potential.

But when we find ways to harness our minds, we can defy all odds. From overcoming depression, abuse, financial strain, or illness to conquering the most unimaginably lofty goals, when properly vanquished, our minds become the weapon needed for success on any battlefield. We just have to embrace the suck.

About a year ago, Brent asked me to send a few motivational words to one of his mentees who was about to begin SEAL training Hell Week. This young man had lost his mother to a sudden brain aneurysm a week before checking in at the command. This is the message I sent, which was shared with the entire class:

> Please tell him that my words will make no difference when his balls are in his stomach from being so cold. Men don't get many chances to show their grit! You need to pray for bad weather! Pray for the coldest water! Pray for a broken fucking body! You should want the worst-case scenario for everything you do in Hell Week! Pray for it to be so hard that only your fucking boat crew makes it all the way through! They succeed because you lead those motherfuckers through the worst Hell Week ever!
>
> You have to become the devil to get through Hell! This shit is about your fucking mindset! If you are hoping for the fucking

best-case scenario in Hell Week, you are not ready! Know that no motherfucker can endure what you can. Not because you believe in yourself. But because you have trained harder than any motherfucker alive!

You might think this is a fucking motivational speech! Well it's not! This is my mentality before I go into any fucking war. Hell Week is not for the faint of heart. It's for that motherfucker looking for the beginning of his soul. You want to see where most people end, and you begin. Be that guy; when everyone is in pain and miserable with their heads hanging low, you're the one smiling! Not a friendly smile, but one that says, "You think this fucking shit can hurt me?!"

This is your time to start creating the person you want to be! You can't make that man in a soft fucking environment! You must be willing to suffer more than anyone else! Not because you have to, but because you want to!

I leave you with this: many people are looking for hard shit so they can prove themselves, but once the hard shit comes, the reality is too much to bear. Be watching for "the look"! You will know it once you see it. It's like their soul is leaving their body. It happens during deep suffering, when a person can no longer handle the mental pain and anguish of what they thought they could do. The key word is "thought" they could do! After you see the look, quitting is very near.

So, what the fuck are you going to do when your balls are in your stomach from the cold? What are you going to do when your body is broke as fuck and you have fifty hours left? What are you going to do when your boat crew starts to quit and you feel alone? What are you going to do when it won't stop raining

and you can't get warm? I don't know what you're going to do.
But you asked me for my advice, so here's what the fuck I did: I
prayed to God to make it worse! Mindset!

Go to war with yourself!

We all have it in ourselves to step boldly onto our battlefield
and take the fight to the enemy, to willingly go to war with ourselves, defy the odds, and live our own version of an extraordinary life. Regardless of all the inevitable obstacles we face from
the day we're born until the day we go over the great divide, if we
simply embrace the suck and go all in, there's no limit to what we
can accomplish.

Pain unlocks a secret doorway in the mind, one that leads to
both peak performance and beautiful silence.

So, don your battle gear and get after it. Good luck.

INTRODUCTION

Do not pray for an easy life, pray for the strength to endure a difficult one.

—BRUCE LEE

This is a book about resilience—a valuable weapon many of us across the globe have needed to arm ourselves with over the past year. While the contents of this book are timeless and the tools it provides apply in *any* scenario, its release was unfortunately ironic. The unprecedented pandemic that rocked the world to its core in 2020 has reshaped the context of our current perceptions of just about everything, including our priorities, health, families, businesses, finances, faith, and love. Developing resilience largely depends on our ability to change the narrative in our minds around the inevitable challenges we face in life and find new answers to these important questions:

What do I consider to be true adversity?

How long do I wallow in my misery?

Are emotional and physical pain realities to be avoided or embraced?

How often do I dwell on things out of my control?

How quickly do I bounce back?

Am I willing to embrace extreme discomfort to live my extraordinary life?

We are the architects of our own beliefs, the decisions we make, and the results those decisions deliver. We may not always realize it, but we have a relatively significant impact on how our lives unfold. The most mentally and physically tough people I know constantly practice the fine art of building resilience—deliberately pounding away at the boundaries of their comfort zone in pursuit of their passions and causes greater than themselves. Simply put, they choose adversity over mediocrity and continue pushing forward despite the odds stacked against them.

> If you can't fly then run, if you can't run then walk,
> if you can't walk then crawl, but whatever you do
> you have to keep moving forward.
>
> —MARTIN LUTHER KING JR.

In early 2000, I made a decision that carried lifelong impact. I left a relatively lucrative job as a financial analyst with a global real estate development company to join the United States Navy. The objective? To successfully navigate what is arguably the most challenging special operations training and selection program in the world and become a Navy SEAL. Little did I know that the following months and years would change my perception of adversity forever.

In the coming pages, I will share some of my experiences from SEAL training, combat, business, and life in general. But the fundamental intention of this book is to uncover what really drives us to thrive in adversity. How do we develop resilience? Do some people have larger sums in their resilience bank accounts than others? How can we make more deposits than withdrawals? Does it happen naturally over time or must we train ourselves in the art of mental toughness? The overarching answer is simple. Resilience is like any muscle. With focus and determination—and some of the tools in this book—you can strengthen your mind to overcome any obstacle, crush goals, dominate your battlefield, and live an extraordinary life.

I attribute much of my success in embracing the unimaginable rigors of the SEAL training course to my mentor. My parents both completed their undergraduate education at Southern Methodist University in Dallas, Texas, where I also attended college many years later. When I finally gained the courage to present my parents with this radical and risky strategy of becoming a warrior (instead of a financial analyst) my dad introduced me to one of his close friends and swim teammates from SMU. He graduated, joined the Navy, and became a SEAL during the Vietnam War. He was living in La Jolla, California, just thirty minutes from where I would hopefully one day begin my transformation from tadpole to frogman at the Naval Special Warfare

Center in Coronado, California. My dad figured that his friend might have some wisdom to share, or more accurately, the ability to talk me out of it! Time would tell.

Now, many years later, in an effort to continue my service and give back to the Naval Special Warfare (NSW) community, I mentor young people through the program. When I first began mentoring these eager and determined young men, the questions were the same ones I had when I was in their shoes. *What's the hardest part? How did you get through it? Is it more mental or physical? What's the best way to train for this program?* Keep in mind, when I was in college, I placed Navy SEALs on the highest of pedestals. They were untouchable demigods who breathed fire, ate glass, and easily bench pressed five hundred pounds—all while carrying a machine gun and Viking drinking horn full of ale. Their steely-eyed glare alone could put a man six feet under.

Before investing my limited time in being a mentor and knowing most of these young men might fail in their attempt, I needed a process for selecting candidates. I had to uncover the answers to a few key questions: *Which of these guys have the grit to get it done? How do I determine who has the appropriate level of resilience? Why do some spend years preparing only to quit on day one while others crush the training with a smile on their face?* So, I asked a high-ranking SEAL commander and fellow board member of the SEAL Family Foundation if NSW had conducted any research to define the mental, emotional, cognitive, and physical attributes of the candidates who are most likely to graduate the course. The pipeline is well over a year of extremely demanding training, and it carries an attrition rate that scares most off before they even sign up. It's very competitive just to be accepted into the program, much less graduate and be welcomed into "the brotherhood." And of those highly capable students who begin, only about 15 percent earn their Trident pin and go to a team. Oh, and then the training regime (and lifestyle) becomes even more taxing, but we'll come back to that.

His response was that NSW had in fact invested significant resources in this research. What he then told me might not be the initial response most would expect—a narrative about star athletes, academic excellence, and brutes who have a penchant for kicking ass and taking names. Obviously, athleticism and intellect play a role, but it's far deeper than these attributes alone: grit, resilience, and a deep passion to serve as a SEAL rank at the top. Essentially, the consistent data and "recipe" for success is reflected in the opening paragraph of the Navy SEAL Ethos, which ironically wasn't created until 2005:

In times of war or uncertainty there is a special breed of warrior ready to answer our nation's call. A common man with uncommon desire to succeed. Forged by adversity, he stands alongside America's finest special operations forces to serve his country, the American people, and protect their way of life. I am that man.

A common man with uncommon desire to succeed. Forged by adversity. Upon further reflection, I boiled what the commander told me down into what I now refer to as The Three Ps: **Persistence, Purpose, and Passion.**

That's it. Sure, you won't even be accepted into the course unless you're in peak physical condition and meet the academic standards. But none of that matters in the first few weeks of Basic Underwater Demolition/SEAL (BUD/S), which kick off a long and arduous journey. Achieving any lofty goal or overcoming life's seemingly insurmountable challenges require persistence, purpose, and passion. The Three Ps aid in the necessary emotional connection for high levels of achievement, be it becoming a Navy SEAL, getting into Harvard, or beating cancer.

I am currently the founder and CEO of TakingPoint Leadership. We partner with our clients on leadership and organizational development initiatives to help them create cultures of high performance. One of the learning modules in our leadership development program is on cultivating resilience in ourselves and others. We break the definition of resilience into three categories:

1. **Challenge:** Resilient people view difficulty as a challenge, not as a paralyzing event. They look at their failures and mistakes as lessons to be learned from and opportunities for growth. In our words, they embrace the suck better than others because they lean in.

2. **Commitment:** Resilient people are committed to their lives and goals. They have a compelling reason to get out of bed in the morning. They are not easily deterred or distracted by "opportunities" that are unrelated to their desired outcomes.

3. **Control:** Resilient people spend their time and energy focusing on situations and events that they have control over. And because they put their efforts where they can have the most impact, they feel empowered and confident.

We also teach Carol S. Dweck's philosophies on *growth* versus *fixed* mindset. Dweck is the Lewis and Virginia Eaton professor of psychology at Stanford University, and she is known for her work on the mindset psychological trait. She taught at Columbia University, Harvard University, and the University of Illinois before joining the Stanford faculty in 2004. According to Dweck, in a growth mindset, people believe that their most basic abilities can be developed through dedication and hard work—brains and talent are just the starting point. This view creates a love of learning and a resilience that is essential for great accomplishment.

Growth and fixed mindsets can be further broken down into five categories: Skills, Challenges, Effort, Feedback, Setbacks.

FIXED MINDSET		GROWTH MINDSET
• Something you're born with • Can't improve	SKILLS	• A result of hard work • Can always improve
• Something to avoid • Could reveal lack of skill • Tend to give up easily	CHALLENGES	• Should be embraced • Provide an opportunity to grow • Produce persistence
• Won't drive desired results • Only for combating inadequacy	EFFORT	• Essential • A path to mastery
• Causes defensiveness • Trend toward taking it personally	FEEDBACK	• Imperative • Critical for learning • Identify areas to improve
• Place blame on others • Result in discouragement	SETBACKS	• A wake-up call • Opportunity for course correction

When we become trapped by a *fixed mindset*, we believe our skills are essentially defined at birth. Challenges are to be avoided at all costs. Feedback is taken personally as opposed to viewed as useful data to learn from. Setbacks are based on external factors and result in discouragement.

A *growth mindset* is the bedrock of resilience. With a growth mindset you know that skills and success come from hard work and dedication, and the status quo is never enough. People with this mindset are comfortable being uncomfortable. Transparent feedback is not just accepted but craved, and setbacks are just another bump in the road fueling the fire to push forward.

A growth mindset is essential for embracing the pain and misery of SEAL training and high performance in any endeavor. It's also critical for embracing the suck life throws at us when we least expect it, and essential for accomplishment and dominating *any* battlefield. When I was at SMU, I was a member of the Phi Gamma Delta fraternity. I know what you're thinking, but just bear with me. We held our weekly meeting every Monday night after dinner in a private room on the third floor of the fraternity house. Each night, without fail, we closed the meeting by reciting a famous quote on the value of persistence from former President Calvin Coolidge.

Nothing in this world can take the place of persistence. **Talent** will not: nothing is more common than unsuccessful men with talent. **Genius** will not: unrewarded genius is almost a proverb. **Education** will not: the world is full of educated derelicts. Persistence and determination alone are omnipotent.

So, many years later, with a few impactful life lessons under my belt, I embarked on my mentorship journey to find only the young men with the most persistence, purpose, and passion. The ones who were not only willing to embrace the suck, but *longed* for it. This isn't easy to measure, especially before BUD/S students are truly tested by the infamous and brutal crucible that goes by the appropriate moniker of *Hell Week*. But by asking the right questions and better understanding their purpose, I have been able to choose mentees who have what it takes. And all of them, so far, have become SEALs. I am in no way taking credit for their success. The grit they needed to see it through came purely from within.

Interestingly, none of them have been college track stars or Olympic swimmers. But they each had a personal connection to the mission and a deep passion around the idea of military service at the most elite level. That connection and passion has continued to drive their resilience in the worst of times. My most recent mentee has had an oddly similar journey to mine, with one exception. He grew up in Rancho Santa Fe, California, five minutes from where I currently live, graduated from college, and began a career in finance only to shift his focus to become a NSW warrior. Sound familiar? Then, the most horrible and unforeseen event occurred. As David mentioned in the foreword, one week before he checked in for BUD/S, his mother died suddenly of a brain aneurysm. Undeterred, and with a new pain to use as fuel for his journey, he dominated the training pipeline and received orders to SEAL Team Three. He became a frogman, well-equipped to take the fight to the enemy.

Nothing great in this world comes without a little bit of adversity. Nothing amazing happens inside our comfort zones. Whether we are talking about getting a promotion, nurturing a challenged marriage, mastering a sport, building or saving a small business, navigating a pandemic, battling disease, dealing with the loss of a loved one, raising children, or hunting terrorists, a little bit of suffering will always be attached. That's why the things we love and work hard for are deeply rewarding. My hope is that this book will provide you with the ammunition and inspiration necessary to embrace the suck, keep fighting, and live an extraordinary life.

PART 1

EMBRACE THE SUCK

We must embrace pain and burn it as fuel for our journey.

—KENJI MIYAZAWA

1
PAIN IS A PATHWAY

Pain is inevitable. Suffering is optional.

—BUDDHIST PROVERB

Al Fallujah, Iraq
1:37 A.M.

You never forget the stench of a war zone, a place full of pain and suffering for all involved.

Our small convoy of Humvees rolled slowly through the rural neighborhood. Each operator was intensely alert, scanning for enemy threats around every corner and on every rooftop. We had turned off the headlights and were driving *blacked out*, using night vision goggles (NVGs). Five minutes earlier, our assault force had met at a predetermined *set point* about half a mile from where our high value target (HVT) was apparently holed up in a two-story house in an upscale area outside the city. We had four vehicles full of SEAL operators and a black Suburban SUV carrying agency partners, the source who had provided the intelligence, and an

Army Ranger unit acting as our blocking force (they would cordon off the area so no one could move in or out).

Each vehicle had two SEALs standing on both port and starboard running boards carrying ladders, with additional assaulters in the back, ready for a quick dismount. I was on the port side of Vehicle 2 holding on to a nylon strap fastened to the roof with my right hand, left hand clutching the side of a wooden ladder. My M4 rifle was strapped tight across my chest. The green haze of my NVGs cast a surreal depiction of the surrounding environment. We were skeptical about the intel because the source seemed nervous and had changed his story several times. We were all on high alert.

The breaks squealed as the convoy rolled to a stop and we quickly dismounted. "The house is fifty meters up the road on the right," our platoon commander said over the radio. The assault team dismounted while our drivers and gunners trailed behind us ready to act as a quick reaction force if the op went sideways. We silently shuffled down the dirt road, eight of us carrying the ladders so we could scale the wall the source said surrounded the house, while the others covered our approach. We slowed as we came to the corner of the lot and noticed something odd. "What the hell? There's no wall in front of the house," one of our point men said in a loud whisper. "Ditch the ladders."

We filed into a perfectly assembled assault train as he led us toward the main entrance. The place looked like a small fortress, not a traditional home. Side by side, two point men crept to the door as the team stacked against the outer wall. One tried the handle. "Locked. Explosive breach," he said.

He pulled a bundle of C-4 explosive from his kit and prepped the charge, while the second SEAL held his rifle pointed at the door. I waited with the rest of the team, sweat already pouring down my back from the humidity and heavy gear. When the charge was fixed to the door, they quickly moved back to our position. "Charge is set. Three, two, one. Execute."

BOOM!

The breaching charge blew the door into three pieces and sent thick chunks of burning wood and metal flying in all directions. We surged through the smoldering entryway. Out of the smoke, a bear of a man came charging straight for us. The first three guys in the stack immediately opened fire, zipping him up with several rounds from their suppressed short barrel M4 rifles. As is the case with most enemy targets in the Middle East, there were multiple noncombatants, women, and children in the house. Two rounds passed through the man's right side and hit his wife in the hip. We can't render medical aid until the fight is won, so we had to keep pressing forward, each SEAL stepping over the massive body and peeling right and left into the compound. The house looked nothing like the source had described. Instead of being in a front living room, we found ourselves in a large open courtyard surrounded by a two-story building with multiple rooms on both levels. We were immediately spread thin, and with shots fired, this was now a *hot target*. Two SEALs and I moved right across the southwest corner of the courtyard toward an open door. An unarmed military-aged male emerged and moved toward us frantically. My teammate struck him in the chest with the muzzle of his suppressed rifle, sending him crumbling to the floor. I pounced on him, quickly pulling thick plastic flex cuffs from my kit and using them to secure his wrists behind his back.

Our chief was directing traffic. "Leave him. Keep clearing the south side," he said. I moved swiftly toward the open door, weapon pointed directly at the entrance. I shifted to the left across the doorway, scanning as much of the room as I could before entering. I moved to the side of the entrance and waited for the shoulder squeeze that signaled that a teammate was ready to move in with me. But there was no squeeze; everyone was dealing with other threats. A man emerged from the darkness with an AK-47 pointed right at me. From the doorway, I took immediate action, placing two rounds in the center of his chest followed by one at the base of his nose. His momentum carried him as he fell to the ground at my feet. I flipped my night vision goggles up onto my helmet and looked down. His bottom jaw was severed completely. He couldn't have been more than nineteen. *What the fuck, you stupid son of a bitch!?* I was livid. Why did he have to force my hand?

A few minutes later, the target was secure, and we began our search for additional intel. Our corpsman immediately began providing medical aid to the woman, while another SEAL got on the radio to call in the medevac helicopter. We loaded the dead combatants into body bags and placed them in the back of one of the vehicles. The next day we received word that the woman lived.

Back at base later that night, I buried my face in my pillow, consumed with pain and confusion. I reflected on the early stages of my SEAL training—how horrific it was and how much resilience I needed to navigate the physical and emotional challenges we faced each day. At the time, we didn't know that the evil bitch of war was lurking just around the bend, which would require a whole new level of fortitude.

What drives resilience in each of us is very personal. Our passions and purpose are a culmination of varying events, experiences, beliefs, values, and external factors. Norman Garmezy, a developmental psychologist and clinician at the University of Minnesota, met thousands of children in his four decades of research. But one nine-year-old, with an alcoholic, schizophrenic mother and an absent father, particularly stood out. Each day, he'd show up to school with the same sandwich in a brown paper bag: two slices of bread with nothing in between. The reality was that there was no other food available and nobody at home competent enough to provide other options. Even so, the boy didn't want people to pity him or know just how grim his situation was. Every day, without fail, he would show up with a smile on his face and a brown bag of bread tucked under one arm.

The boy with the bread sandwich was part of a special group of children. He belonged to a cohort of kids—the first of many—whom Garmezy would go on to identify as succeeding, even excelling, despite incredibly difficult circumstances. These were the children who exhibited a trait Garmezy would later identify as *resilience*. He is now widely credited with being the first to study the concept in an experimental setting. Over many years, Garmezy visited schools across the country, focusing on those in economically depressed areas, and followed a standard protocol. He would set up meetings with the principal, along with a school social worker or nurse, and pose the same question: *Were there any children whose backgrounds had initially raised red flags—kids who seemed likely to become problem children—who had instead become, surprisingly, a source of pride for the school?* Garmezy said, in a 1999 interview, "If I had said, 'Do you have kids in this school who seem to be troubled?' there wouldn't have been a moment's delay. But to be asked about children who were adaptive and good citizens—who excelled even though they came from very disturbed backgrounds—that was a new sort of inquiry. That's the way we began."

Resilience presents a challenge for many psychologists. Whether you can be said to have it or not largely depends not on any particular psychological test but on the way your life unfolds. If you are lucky (or unlucky) enough to never experience any sort of adversity, you won't know how resilient you are. It's only when you're faced with obstacles, stress, and other environmental threats that resilience, or the lack of it, emerges. Do you succumb, or do you surmount?

Somewhere in Hell
March 2001, Coronado, California
12:04 A.M.

I gasped violently as my head re-emerged from the icy froth of the fifty-five-degree surf zone. A perfect cocktail of saltwater and mucus streamed from my nostrils and down onto my lips and chin. My sinuses and eyes burned from being constantly purged by the Pacific Ocean. The cascading headlights from the two white Ford F-150 pickup trucks pointed in our direction were blinding. I looked up for a brief moment and noticed the warm glow coming from a few of the cozy condominiums stacked in the tall white towers looming over us. The briny smell of ocean water lingered in the cold night air.

BUD/S class 235 was a mere four hours into Hell Week, the brutal crucible that weeds most students out of the Navy SEAL training and selection program. We were lying in the surf zone, arms linked, feet toward the beach. We shivered uncontrollably in our wonderful human chain of miserable convulsions. The instructors had ordered a round of "rocking chairs." The class lies down together in about a foot of water, and in unison everyone kicks their legs back up and over their heads. Back and forth, back and forth until the instructors have had enough. This exercise forces your head underwater at a downward angle shooting cold seawater into your sinus cavity.

We were clad in green, brown, and black jungle camo battle dress uniforms (BDUs), black Bates tactical sport boots, orange life vests, and black Pro-Tec helmets. I had a hairline fracture in my left elbow that was causing severe swelling due to bursitis, overuse injuries to the iliotibial bands in both legs, and a flesh-eating bacteria snacking away at my right calve. Oh, and did I mention it was fucking raining? It rarely rains in San Diego. It was glorious. Everything was coming together nicely. The good Lord needs dangerous frogmen, which can only be forged in adversity. David Goggins's prayers had been answered. As the Navy SEAL Ethos states, "My Nation expects me to be physically harder and mentally stronger than my enemies." One of the instructors standing over us said something I'll never forget, "Gentlemen, take all that pain, shaking, and cold and turn it into aggression. Let it drive you."

Four hours earlier, Hell Week *breakout* had commenced. Once you've been through about a month of indoctrination and a few weeks of the first phase of the BUD/S program, you arrive at Hell Week. And it is exactly what it sounds like. At this point, about half the class has already quit. And many more will ring the bell during the first couple days. The weeks leading up to this period are no picnic either. Most of the class enters Hell Week either sick or having sustained multiple injuries. Or both.

So when the agony is getting ready to start on a Sunday evening, you're already miserable with anticipation. The group reports to the main classroom on Sunday morning with only a few required items. The beauty of that first day is that you still have no idea exactly when the fun will commence. The stress and anxiety are eating away at the core of your soul, and then suddenly break-out starts. It's a whirlwind of explosions, instructors swarming around you, firing M60 machine guns—using blanks, but still. You're getting sprayed with fire hoses, and smoke grenades are going off everywhere. For the residents of the high-rise condo towers just up the beach it looks like a fierce battle has broken out.

The instructors are shouting orders. "Bear crawl to the surf zone—get wet and sandy!" "Boat crew leaders, give me a head-count!" "One hundred burpees! Bust 'em out!" It's total chaos. After a couple hours of insanity, the class heads to the beach for "surf torture." Similar to rocking chairs, you link arms with your classmates and walk into the ocean and lie down. Unlike the fire and brimstone of actual hell, the instructors want to make sure they keep you extremely cold, wet, and sandy all week. My class had the privilege of enduring Hell Week in the winter, when water temps in Coronado can be in the fifties. And you know what? Fantastic. The mindfuck of being freezing cold and soaking wet twenty-four hours a day is what drives most students to throw in the towel.

It's not uncommon for students to quit even in the first few hours. I enjoyed watching others drop on request (DOR) because I knew it meant my chances of making it kept improving, statis-tically speaking. For six days, you won't have more than a cou-ple hours of sleep. Even when you are allowed to sleep it's not exactly restful. Whenever you stop moving, your muscles cramp up uncontrollably—the pain is overwhelming and you can't even fathom being able to move again. But you quickly learn that the mind can be a powerful tool when harnessed properly.

Everything about Hell Week is designed to test your physical and mental fortitude. You're running and crawling everywhere, covered in sand, flesh sloughing off as you go. You run the equivalent of multiple marathons. Swim dozens of miles in the frigid ocean. Run carrying heavy logs, boats, and backpacks. And everything is a race. If you're not "putting out," the instructors hammer your ass. That is, if your boat crew doesn't tune you up first. It's nonstop intense physical activity, and the instructors are whispering in your ear every minute, trying to get you to quit.

"Gleeson, come on man. This isn't for you. You're not cut out for this. Hop in the truck—we have blankets and hot coffee." They are like the sirens from Greek mythology luring sailors to their watery demise, and guys fall for it all the time. But an hour later, when they're warm and dry, all they know is the fierce sting of regret.

You only stop moving to eat. That could mean running over to the chow hall or eating a cold Meal, Ready-to-Eat (MRE) in the surf zone. Some of us started putting the MRE water-activated meal heaters inside our shirts for a brief moment of warmth. When the instructors caught wind of this, they made us relinquish all meal heaters for the rest of the week. Naughty BUD/S students!

What gets you through is your mindset, resolve, and the leadership of the officers in the class. And, of course, The Three Ps. Our class leader—the highest-ranking officer—was the ideal combination of tough, principled, and compassionate. We all gravitated toward John. He had a positive mental attitude and an innate ability to fire us up about the misery we would face each day. On Sunday afternoon, as fear consumed us in the classroom, he read us the St. Crispin's Day speech from William Shakespeare's *Henry V*. This speech has a lot of meaning to me. I was the captain of our rugby team my junior and senior years at SMU, and we had an excerpt from it printed on the back of our team T-shirts.

John read aloud those famed lines: *"From this day to the ending of the world, but we in it shall be remembered. We few, we happy few, we band of brothers; For he today that sheds his blood with me shall be my brother."*

John died four days later—he drowned in the pool after suffering from severe pulmonary edema. He was laid to rest at Fort Rosecrans National Cemetery and will forever be my brother. It was my first Navy funeral—I had no idea it would be the first of so many. His Hell Week boat paddle hangs on the wall in my office. I offered it to his family, but they politely declined. It's a monument to the extreme sacrifices men will make just attempting to serve as a SEAL—a goal, when successfully achieved, that only leads to greater sacrifice.

So, after a seemingly endless session of surf torture, our first evolution of the night was *rock portage*. We paddled our black rubber boats out through the powerful eight-foot waves turning north to head up the beach toward the famous Hotel del Coronado. That part alone was the cause of severe injury for a few of our classmates. If your timing is off or the crew out of synch, the crashing waves can launch an entire boat backward, sending BUD/S students flying in all directions like rag dolls at the mercy of the dark sea.

> The fishermen know that the sea is dangerous and the storm terrible, but they have never found these dangers sufficient reason for staying ashore.
>
> —VINCENT VAN GOGH

To the casual observer from the beach, this might look either horrifying or hilarious depending on your psychological makeup. What one might not see from a distance, however, is oar handles smashing in teeth, elbows cracking cheek bones, a classmate's helmet breaking his buddy's nose, muscle-bound men landing on top of each other, and boats trapping students underwater for what seems like an eternity.

Why were we paddling up to the Hotel del Coronado? Let's just say it wasn't for cocktails with pink umbrellas or spa treatments consisting of a massage, facial, and body wrap. (Although the sand in my pants was doing a wonderful job of exfoliation ... just a couple layers of skin too deep.) If you've ever been to The Del, you may recall the massive jagged rock formation that sprawls seventy-five yards along the beach just in front of the southernmost part of the hotel. It's as if God Himself, in all His mischievous glory, reached down and strategically placed each giant boulder purely for the sake of SEAL training—nothing else but flat white sand for miles on either side. We had spent the preceding weeks running and swimming up past the formation and back while performing our four-mile runs and two-mile ocean swims, which required more competitive minimum times as you progressed through each phase of BUD/S.

During rock portage, the instructors have a sensational skill for timing the surf just right so that the waves are at their max, crashing so violently against the rock face you can hear it from every room in the hotel. The goal of rock portage is to paddle through the surf, land your 250-pound boat on the rocks, and successfully carry it up and over onto the beach—with each boat crew member present and accounted for. To the passerby during the day, the rocks may not look all that intimidating—with jovial youngsters climbing around and happy couples snapping selfies for Instagram. But to the BUD/S students in the water, with high surf at nighttime, they look like the cliffs surrounding Kalaupapa on the Hawaiian island of Moloka'i. Just Google it, you'll get the idea.

My boat crew, Boat Crew 2, floated just beyond the surf zone waiting for what felt like the right moment. Each boat carries six enlisted students and one officer—the crew leader. Included in my crew was David Goggins and Drew Sheets—two of the toughest guys I'd ever met. Pistachio-size raindrops were ricocheting off our helmets and the hard rubber frame of the boat. The clouds had parted just enough to allow a beam of moonlight to guide our path to potential destruction. It was like a well-lit runway—but at the end of the runway was annihilation. The only source of moderate warmth came from the rigors of paddling the boat and the occasional peeing in one's pants. Yes, you read that correctly; the warm urine provided ten seconds of extraordinary bliss. It's the little pleasures in life, right?

"Now! Paddle!" our boat crew leader suddenly shouted. We surged forward at an aggressive yet somewhat cautious pace, trying to time the waves just right. If the surf was too low, we'd land at the bottom of the rocks and get crushed when larger waves came in on top of us as we ascended. If it was too high, we could lose control of the boat and be flung into the rocks at bone-crushing velocity.

We rode a medium-sized wave in, positioning the front of the boat on the edge of one of the larger boulders. Two of us leapt out, holding the lines so we could keep the boat steady and upright. Amid the struggle, I looked to my right and saw one of my friends get tossed from his boat as it hit the rocks. He landed head and shoulders down in a crevice between two rocks, only his waist and legs above water. I later found out he almost drowned and ended up with a broken arm and fractured collarbone. But there was nothing I could do for him. I had my own crew to worry about. We hauled our boat up and over the rocks to the safe embrace of SEAL instructors ready to dole out some more pain.

The hotel guests with a lust for late-night socializing often come out to watch the fun unfold. The instructors, injured students (also known as "roll backs"), and Navy corpsmen had the area blocked off with yellow tape and orange cones, making it look like a crime scene. For the participants, it felt like one too. The only difference was that we had actually volunteered for this punishment. Two of the hotel guests that evening were my parents. They weren't there to socialize; they'd come to watch their baby boy suffer. My mom would later describe the moment as one of sheer horror. She only watched for a few minutes before retreating to the blissful denial of their luxury hotel room, 1,200-thread count sheets and all. I don't blame her. She couldn't even bear to watch my college rugby games because of the injuries I sustained during my first two matches.

Another hidden gem from this evolution is the extremely porous nature of the rocks—similar to a sharp coral. Due to adrenaline, you don't realize it at the time, but as you crawl over the rocks straining to carry the heavy boat, the tiny razor-sharp edges are shredding your hands and wrists. Your water-soaked flesh is already soft and vulnerable. The aftermath looks like an evil forest fairy with a vengeance wielding a tiny ice cream scoop went to town on your skin. Small, deep, bloody pockmarks remain. Many have those scars for years to come.

✪

"Gentlemen, take all that pain, shaking, and misery and turn it into aggression. Let it drive you," the instructor said calmly into his megaphone.

I snapped out of it—I was still lying in the surf zone doing rocking chairs. And then the most unimaginably morose feeling swept over me. This incomprehensible pain was going to last twenty-four hours a day until Friday afternoon. And it would only get worse as the week went on. Home seemed like a distant memory.

Light at the end of the tunnel? Not even a tiny fucking glimmer.

Assuming you don't live in a cave shielded from all of the suffering life throws at you (although living in a cave would still suck), I'm sure this has happened to you: you try to comprehend a difficult situation, but in the moment your brain just doesn't get it. Like when I tell our oldest son to stop playing *Fortnite* and do his chores.

In that moment, I quickly learned a fabulously simple solution:

Just give up.

Don't fight it.

Embrace the pain.

Beg for more.

Change the narrative in your mind.

If you're struggling to wrap your head around an uncomfortable situation, then the following happens: As soon as your brain receives input, the synapses start to fire their little electrons and look for pre-existing structures to attach your new input to—such as hypothermia, bone fractures, and flesh-eating bacteria. But in this case, there just isn't any place for the electrons to attach because the input is new, shitty, and unfamiliar—it doesn't quite fit anywhere. Then your brain becomes sad, very sad. The new input is like sand in your hands. Or in this case, covering your entire body. Your brain just lets it trickle through—comprehension becomes a challenge.

In that moment, the *Embrace the Suck* philosophy was born. I not only gave in to my reality, I embraced it. It was exhilarating (maybe it was just my drunken state of hypothermia, but you get the idea). As I laid in the surf next to my brothers, shivering violently, I reminded myself that I had chosen this. I had sacrificed everything—a good job, nice apartment, time with friends and family—and had to crush the boundaries of my comfort zone just to be accepted into the program. This was *purposeful suffering*. It had meaning. There was a vision. A call to serve. If I didn't lean into it, all would be lost.

Suck it the fuck up. You earned your right to be here. You have a long way to go, so embrace the suck and get it done.

Those of us that embraced this mindset succeeded in our endeavor.

Mental Model

The Pain Transformation Process

Psychologists who have studied victims of severe physical and emotional trauma have found that while individuals who have experienced great pain and suffering aren't exactly thrilled about it, the vast majority feel they have grown substantially from those experiences. Many claim to have gained an eye-opening perspective on life and become more responsible, more resilient, less self-absorbed, and even happier.

Polish psychologist Kazimierz Dąbrowski argues that fear, anxiety, and sadness are not always undesirable or damaging states of mind, but rather representative of the necessary pain for psychological growth. To avoid pain is basically to deny our own potential. You don't build muscle or physical stamina without experiencing pain. But it's the type of pain that signifies forward progress. Similarly, we can't develop psychological resilience without experiencing emotional pain and suffering.

And let's just say you don't reach peak mental and physical toughness without embracing a whole lot of suck. As the famed Marine Corps officer Chesty Puller said, "Pain is weakness leaving the body."

This saying is revered by rugby players worldwide. Before games, I used to find a private place, take a Buck hunting knife I'd received for Christmas as a kid (yes, that's what you get for Christmas in Texas), and cut my thigh—I'd rub the blood on my face to prepare for battle. Then I'd tape up the wound and head out to the field to warm up. I know what you're thinking. *Brent, what the hell is wrong with you?!* If I didn't leave the rugby field with a significant injury—or if I failed to inflict pain on the foe—I would berate myself for not playing hard enough. Eight concussions, three shattered teeth, and one Hell Week later, I found out that my tolerance for (or maybe enjoyment of) pain would serve me well.

Becoming more resilient starts with changing your perspective on adversity. Pain can in fact be transformed into a useful energy force for accomplishing great feats. For gaining perspective. For building physical and emotional resilience. When you can master the ability to control pain whatever form it comes in—and even lean into it, it doesn't have to hurt so badly.

Pain Don't Hurt

I don't usually look to the late Patrick Swayze for life advice, but his role as Dalton in the '80s film *Road House* embodies this mindset perfectly. Dalton is a PhD-educated, karate ass-kicking, professional bouncer brought in to transform a local bar. Kind of like the hit TV show *Bar Rescue*, I guess. Dalton is what's called a "cooler," a specialized bouncer with a mysterious past who is lured from his job at a club in New York City to take over security at a nightclub in Jasper, Missouri, the wild and raucous Double Deuce. But a corrupt local businessman isn't having it and sends his goons in to take back control.

Dalton has been in yet another knife fight at his new place of business and heads to the hospital for stitches. In walks the doctor. She's wearing a white lab coat, has big bangs and an aggressive blonde perm. She examines his many scars with a confused frown, then asks if he wants a local anesthetic.

In a southern accent he says, "No thank you, ma'am." She then asks him, "Do you like pain, Mr. Dalton?" His famous response: "Pain don't hurt."

Pain, sorrow, and tragedy—like getting stabbed by an angry drunkard in a crappy bar—are not what we seek out in life. But much of life's suffering is inevitable. The more readily we lean into pain, loss, and disappointment the sooner we will learn how to gain from these experiences and move forward. Of course, there are certain experiences we'll never truly embrace, such as the death of a parent, friend, child, or spouse. But there are ways to celebrate life and still find happiness in times of loss. And it's not about the pain itself but rather how and why we choose to suffer. And most importantly, what we can potentially gain from it. More on that in Chapter Seven.

And sometimes, pain and adversity open the door to new opportunities, like meeting a pretty doctor with a bad perm, winning a rugby game, completing Hell Week, accomplishing athletic feats of greatness, transforming a business, defeating our nation's enemies, landing your dream job, or finding the love of your life.

Let me ask you this. When the hell have you ever accomplished anything spectacular while nestled safely in your comfort zone?

We both know the answer. Never.

We all know today's culture has a fascination with risk-takers and we crave motivational social media posts that keep our head in the game. Like when David Goggins makes you realize you're a wimp who complains about dumb shit! We also know that our openness to taking some risk (not blind dumb risk, but calculated risk) directly correlates to new possibilities and a bright future. Yet what do we often do? We stay comfortable in our safe little world living vicariously through other more daring beings.

Why? Because the very instincts we humans once needed to avoid the pain of being devoured by a saber-toothed cat or attacked by a band of marauding warriors are the same that keep us from taking new risks. Venturing out. Trying new things. Getting out there in that big scary world and saying fuck it. Saying yes to life. The good, the bad, and the ugly.

But guess what: the world isn't actually as scary as it was a long time ago. Sure, the world is, and always will be, a place of needless violence and suffering. War will always exist. Foreign and domestic terrorism isn't going anywhere anytime soon. Global pandemics will take lives and businesses. But for most, the likelihood of experiencing the horrors of old, such as being keelhauled by pirates, burned at the stake, stomped to death by a mastodon, or carried away by an angry torch-wielding mob, is quite low.

And while it is part of our universal nature to seek pleasure and avoid pain, culture plays a central role in how we deal with suffering. In the West, we generally reject suffering. We see it as an unwelcome interruption to our pursuit of happiness. So we fight it, repress it, medicate it, or search for quick-fix solutions to get rid of it. In some cultures, especially in the East, suffering is acknowledged for the important role it plays in people's lives on the meandering path toward enlightenment. But the fact that suffering yields benefits does not imply that we ought to seek it actively—sickness strengthens our immune system, but that does not imply that we need to look for opportunities to become sick. We naturally seek pleasure in our lives and try to minimize the amount of pain we endure. Yet it still finds us.

So how do we channel emotional, psychological, and physical pain and use it as a pathway? By following the Pain Is a Pathway mental model.

THE ACT	THE PROCESS
Fully experience your pain and emotions.	The largest mistake people make is masking their emotions and denying their true suffering. This is counterproductive and can lead to deeper problems in the future. When each emotion comes, feel it. Your body will tell you when it's enough. Cry, scream, and cry again—maybe not in public though (or SEAL training). Submit to the beginning of a process that will take time to complete. To feel is to be human, embrace it!
Challenge your perspective.	The downward spiral never lasts forever, hence the saying "This too shall pass." But when it seems the razorblade-covered waterslide to hell has no end, you can still find ways to focus on the positive instead of the negative. Perspective plays a key role in acceptance. Our brains can be evil fuckers—controlling us, distorting our reality. We must take a step back and challenge our existing way of thinking, conduct a "perspective audit," if you will. Ask: What is the root cause of my existing stress and suffering? Is my current perspective realistic? Is it solving any of my challenges? Or could there possibly be a different—and more productive—way of looking at things?
Surround yourself with the right influences.	During these times you'll find out, like I have, that there are some people you can count on and some you can't. Take this opportunity to weed out those in your life who may be holding you back. Find inspiration in a mentor or someone you love or admire. Lean on family and friends. If you don't have anyone to lean on, reach out to a therapist. If that doesn't work, focus on building new positive relationships. But for God's sake, cut the negative losers from your life who don't wish you well.

THE ACT	THE PROCESS
Stay (or become) active and avoid negative coping mechanisms.	It's useless to focus all your energy on events that you no longer have control over. Instead of wasting time in this way, get active in your everyday life. Take up distance running, swimming, biking, martial arts, or all of the above. And commit to it. Physical and mental wellness are crucial for embracing the suck. Meanwhile, if you are dealing with depression, sadness, or anger, stay away from alcohol and other substances that will only magnify your pain. You may think you are drowning your sorrows, but you're really providing them with fuel. But that's not the kind of fuel you need for your journey.
Know that bad things don't actually come in threes (not sure I totally believe this yet).	Sure, maybe you woke up today with your downstairs bathroom flooding the entire bottom floor only to open your email and read a message from your largest client that they are canceling their contract. Then later, at your annual checkup your doctor tells you that you may have prostate cancer. You're like, "What the fuck?! Seriously?!" Scientists found the reason why bad things "come in threes": they simply don't. We look for patterns in random data as a way to extract order from disorder. This is called confirmation bias—the tendency to favor information that confirms our assumptions, preconceptions, or hypotheses whether or not they are actually and independently true. Our need to find patterns and make sense of everything can distort reality.
Accept and forgive.	Holding on to hatred and resentment—for ourselves or others—only poisons you. Hatred for the enemy that killed your teammate, an ex-spouse and her attorney, the drunk driver that took your sister, COVID-19, the IRS, cancer, everything. It keeps you forever trapped in the past, focusing on an element that you're letting define who you are today. Learn to let go. To give up. Give in. When you do, you'll feel the weight lifted and be able to channel the renewed energy into positive new pursuits. This is easier said than done, of course, and it's not something that will happen overnight either. The only way to truly learn to let go is to allow time to heal you. You'll know when you get there.

Accepting that life will eventually knock you hard on your ass is a stepping-stone to growth. Just expect it to happen. Constantly trying to avoid hardship and pain will only prove detrimental to you. Each experience, each moment that you have is precious. Life is short. I challenge you to make the best out of even the worst circumstances. Like me, you may be amazed at the power, wisdom, and strength you gain.

Great, So What Now?

You might be reading this and telling me to go fuck myself, that I haven't been through the kind of suffering you've endured. And that may very well be true. My intention with this book is not to appear that I know it all or have experienced all the hardships life has to offer. I'm simply providing a tool to use in your own way while navigating darkness and uncertainty.

I'll admit, I grew up relatively privileged. I've never been fired from a job, physically abused (other than SEAL training and combat), or threatened with a debilitating illness or injury. Not yet anyway. But I've seen the horror of war-torn countries. I've taken life, up close and personal. I've lost many friends. I still have blood-stained cammies in a Para bag in my garage—the blood isn't mine. I don't remember the last time I slept through the night, I still wake up every half hour or so—apparently that's not normal. I've been through a horrible divorce driven by infidelity and drug use. No, not by me. I was a full-time single parent to a toddler while building two companies for years before meeting my incredible wife. Who knew? I've experienced financial hardship and the extreme stress of business and entrepreneurship. My pet monkey drowned in a cardboard box in Africa. As I write this,

I'm pivoting to save my current company. I've had horrible diarrhea while on missions in Iraq, more than once. So, like you, I've been through some "shit." And I'm sure life has more in store for me.

Anyway, the point is, we all have our own journeys. But pain can be an incredible pathway to living an extraordinary life if used correctly with the right mindset. We just have to embrace the suck along the way.

Questions to ask yourself:

Do I have more of a fixed mindset or a growth mindset?

If I reflect on some of my more physically and emotionally painful experiences, how did I initially react? How long did it take for me to heal? Could I have done things differently?

How do I apply painful experiences to my growth and development?

Am I becoming more resilient, building brain calluses, or continuing to react in the same way to adversity?

What do I do on a regular basis to inject a little positive pain into my life?

When I have been especially resilient, what was true about me?

2

YOU GOT DEALT A BAD HAND— GET OVER IT

In the midst of chaos, there is also opportunity.

—SUN TZU

I don't really play poker. I can think of better ways to spend my time, especially when it comes to pissing my money away. But poker is all about analyzing the odds. Most mediocre players don't understand this, which is why they are fixated on the cards they're dealt. When they lose, which is often, they think, *Damn, I keep getting dealt shitty cards.* They were either unlucky because they still got beat with a good hand or because they never received good cards in the first place. They see no holes in this flawed logic.

Good and bad cards are dealt to all of us in the same proportion over time. Luck tends to even out. Winning with bad cards—in poker as on the battlefield of life—is a skill that anyone can master. In fact, real winners don't believe in luck. Through vision, hard work, preparation, appropriate course correction, and resilience, they make their own luck. Especially when it comes to bouncing back from adversity.

Outside of unavoidable illness and injuries—or worse—successfully finishing BUD/S has nothing to do with luck. The last month of BUD/S, before transitioning to SEAL Qualification Training (SQT—the advanced portion of the pipeline), is spent on San Clemente Island, the southernmost of California's Channel Islands owned and operated by the US Navy. (Also known by SEAL instructors as "the place where nobody can hear you scream.") Let's just say that bad hands get dealt a lot on the island.

The Wheel of Misfortune
September 2001, San Clemente Island, California
11:00 P.M.

We slid quietly over the sides of our black Zodiac boats into the cold dark Pacific about a half mile off the coast of the island. This was our final training exercise (FTX). BUD/S was almost over. The following week we'd graduate and begin SQT. Little did we know the following week would also mark the beginning of two decades of war . . . the Twin Towers would fall in Manhattan. Our world was about to change.

We were clad in dive hoods, black dry suits, and long fins, and our faces were covered in camo paint. We had our Kelty tactical backpacks in dry bags to keep our gear, explosives, and extra ammo from getting wet. Once in the water, the boats pulled back quietly. We floated in our position for about ten minutes watching the shoreline, then sent in our two swimmer scouts to secure the beach.

Once ashore, they signaled us with three quick flashes from a tactical SureFire flashlight—the sign it was safe to bring the rest of the team over the beach. We swam toward the insert point silently kicking our fins, rifles perched atop our buoyant dry bags should we take fire from the beach—carefully maintaining a low profile. When we were in about four feet of water, each man removed his fins and either slung them over his wrist or quickly attached them to his belt with a carabiner. We moved stealthily out of the water and across the beach to our swimmer scouts while scanning in all directions for threats. We were heavily armed shadowy figures gliding over the sand ready to strike fear in the heart of the enemy. Our scouts had found a nice rock formation that allowed for good cover and concealment for the whole team. We set up a security perimeter and began transitioning out of our dry suits— all of us wearing jungle cammies underneath. Within minutes we were ready to move out. During our mission planning process, we'd mapped out the best route to the enemy compound—a small village and weapons cache. The journey would take us several hours, each student carrying about sixty pounds of gear. I was a machine gunner—carrying the M60 and about one thousand rounds of belt-fed 7.62 ammo. So, let's make that about 100 pounds of gear. The first leg of the route involved scaling the cliff that bordered the beach for miles in both directions. Off we went, hot and sweaty while humping, wet and cold while taking short breaks.

At about 3:00 a.m., we arrived at the coordinates where we'd construct several hide sites to observe the enemy target for three days before initiating our assault. We spread the team out along a ridgeline that provided a great vantage point of the compound about one click (one thousand meters) down in the ravine below.

Time was of the essence as the sun would be peaking over the horizon soon. Harsh punishments are doled out if the instructors discover your hide sight. We busted out our shovels and started digging—others began gathering brush and any available material. The terrain on the island doesn't lend well to natural concealment, so we had to get creative using our packs and camo netting. An hour later, we were huddled in our respective hide sites mentally preparing for three days of living in, well, basically a shallow dirt hole. Talk about embracing the suck!

For the next few days we rotated duties for keeping "eyes on"—making hand sketches of the enemy target, notating sentry routines, taking photos, and relaying intel back to the tactical operations center (TOC) using our Special Operations Tactical Video System. I spent my downtime sleeping, dipping Copenhagen, and daydreaming about our graduation. Sounds fun, right? On the night of the third day, we were ready to make our assault. We packed up our gear and broke down the hides.

We spread out into a skirmish line—each man a few meters apart—and moved down the slope toward the compound. About two hundred meters from the target, we transitioned into an L-ambush formation. One element would be the "base" that would soften the target with a violent barrage of fully automatic machine gun fire. The other element would be the "maneuver" that moved in quickly to begin clearing the compound of remaining enemy threats. Once set, we began the onslaught. Speed, surprise, violence of action.

Thwaaaaaaaaaaap! Thwaaaaaaaaaaap! Thwaaaaaaaaaaap!

I was in the base element. We were all lying in the prone position. Hundreds of well-placed rounds ripped through the walls of each structure. My M60 barrel glowed red as hot empty shell casings expelled from the powerful weapon began raining down on us, finding every piece of exposed skin. The best part is when they wiggle their way inside your camo top burning the shit out of you as they roll down your back. I still have the scars to prove it.

"Shift fire, shift fire," the team leader of the maneuver element said over the radio. We continued the barrage, but shifted our angle of fire toward the opposite end of the compound from where the maneuver element would approach. They moved in quickly and began clearing structures, tossing crash grenades into each hut before entering. *Bang! Bang! Bang!* Then our element moved in—right through a fucking cactus field, of course—to assist with clearance. Once the target was secure and all enemy threats eliminated, we set security and started prepping explosives to blow the weapons cache.

"Gleeson, we're ready for the det cord," our squad leader said, telling me to ready the detonation cord used to connect multiple explosive devices. "Roger that, stand by," I replied, quickly digging into my pack. Then digging a little further. Then a bit further. *Fuck! Oh shiiiiiiiit.*

"Gleeson hurry up, bro!" he said again. "Dude, I can't find it. No idea what happened. I know I packed it!" I responded with a nice blend of panic and utter embarrassment. Luckily our philosophy is two is one, one is none. One of the other guys in the squad passed forward the det cord he had packed. We set the charges and moved out of the blast radius.

"Three, two, one. Execute."

BOOOOOOM! The explosion vaporized the wooden structure, sending fragments of plywood soaring into the moonlit sky. We humped out at a rapid pace so we didn't miss the extraction time window. About ten minutes later, we hit the beach and signaled the boats. They immediately signaled back, and we swam out through the surf zone in true frogman fashion (yet still only tadpoles). Once on the boats, the instructors called the mission complete and we headed back to our campus on the other side of the island for the after-action review—a formal military debrief. My serious infraction did not go overlooked.

We succeed and fail as a team. So, when individuals make mistakes, everyone pays the man. Several of us had screwed up or received safety violations. The instructors assembled the class in formation and ordered three of us to the front where the infamous Wheel of Misfortune had been placed.

Okay, so you've seen the show *Wheel of Fortune*, right? Sure you have. You spin the wheel, pick a letter, and try to solve the puzzle or go bankrupt. But on the show, bankruptcy doesn't come with severe physical punishment—you just lose the money you've earned. Now picture a smaller wooden version of the wheel, but each slot you land on offers a prize of torture, like getting wet and sandy or endless push-ups, burpees, star jumps, or other exhausting rewards.

"Gleeson, you're up!" one instructor shouted. I cringed as I spun the wheel. *Pop, pop, pop, pop, pop . . . pop . . . . . pop . . . . pop . . . . pop.* It slowly came to its resting place. One hundred eight-counts. It was the worst of all the exercises, basically burpees on steroids. The class groaned. We'd been dealt a very bad hand for sure. I could feel the eye-daggers shooting into my back.

"Alright, you see the wheel. One hundred eight-count body builders. Bust 'em!" another instructor growled in a Texas accent. "Hooyah, Instructor Smith!" the class shouted at the top of our lungs in unison. Our class leader took count as we busted out each eight-count. But there was a catch. The class was actually fired up and in good spirits. We were basically done with BUD/S. The next day we'd perform class skits where we get to make fun of our instructors' personality flaws, then head back to Coronado. Each student had embraced so much suck that there was literally nothing the instructors could do to break us at that point, and they knew it. Months of psychological and physical punishment had made us harder and mentally tougher than we'd ever been in our lives. And we'd only get harder as the months and years go on. We'd been dealt a bad hand due to very avoidable mistakes. But so what? Was doing one hundred eight-counts our first choice? No. But we'd happily do one thousand if we had to. We had frogman fire flowing through our veins.

Our class laughed and made jokes, taunting the instructors to give us more. "Beat us harder! What else you got? Hooyah! Hooyahhhhhhh!" There was no longer a boundary to our comfort zone. Acceptance of pain was comfortable.

It had become a pathway.

Of the more than 200 students who began in BUD/S class 235, ultimately only 23 of the original students graduated BUD/S and began SQT. With the war now raging in Afghanistan and rumors of conflicts in Iraq, we all knew that we'd be taking the fight to the enemy, and soon. Mindsets rapidly shifted to the reality that we were now wartime SEALs. After earning my Trident, I was assigned to SEAL Team Five based in Coronado, California. That's when the real training began.

There is no hunting like the hunting of man, and those who have hunted armed men long enough and liked it, never care for anything else thereafter.

—ERNEST HEMINGWAY

In November 2002, my task unit was given the final word that we would be heading to Iraq. SEAL Team Three would be part of the initial assault on the Al-Faw Peninsula, then push north with conventional forces. My task unit from Team Five would take over to run "capture or kill" missions in and around Baghdad, Ar Ramadi, and Al Fallujah to be the hunters of bad men.

We'd been given our ticket to The Show, which many thought might be over before it really began. We were wrong.

Iraq 2007
SEAL Team Ten, Two Weeks Before Deploying Home

If you're curious as to what true resilience looks like, keep reading. This is the story of my friend and SEAL brother Jason Redman.

If knocked down, I will get back up every time....
I am never out of the fight.

—NAVY SEAL ETHOS

"One minute out," the call came over the radio. Three helicopters packed with combat-hardened SEAL operators and their Iraqi counterparts were on their final approach to the enemy target in Al Fallujah. They'd been tasked with capturing a high-ranking Al Qaeda leader, a terrorist they'd been hunting the entire deployment. This intel was as good as it was going to get. There was also a general consensus that they could be walking into a shitstorm of a firefight against highly trained terrorists.

As the SEAL assault force commander, Jason was seated in the lead bird, which was about to touch down in the street right in front of the main gate of the compound. We call this "flying onto the X." Speed, surprise, and violence of action are crucial. The team breacher and point man were seated on one side of the helo with Jason and another SEAL on the other. The landing was supposed to position the breacher's door facing the gate for a speedy exit. But as luck would have it, they landed facing the opposite direction. Time was of the essence, so they had to adapt. Jason and another SEAL leapt from the bird and sprinted to the main gate, the rest of the assault force close on their heels, suppressed weapons pointing in all directions scanning for threats. They checked the gate and to their surprise found it was unlocked. The team entered quickly in expert formation, a result of years of training and hundreds of similar combat missions. They stacked along the outer wall of the main building as the breacher worked to open the door. Jason's heart pounded yet he maintained total situational awareness. Each man moved with complete resolve, knowing they might be walking into a barrage of gunfire immediately upon entry. With the door quickly breached, they flooded the large front room. But instead of taking AK-47 rounds to the chest, there was nothing. They continued to clear the target, moving through the main building and smaller surrounding structures. No bad guys. A dry hole as we call it. They did, however, find a massive weapons cache in one of the smaller buildings along the perimeter of the walled compound. Once the target was officially called clear, they set security and began a sensitive sight exploitation (SSE). Jason stood on the front steps of the central building directing traffic as a Spectre gunship circled overhead providing air support.

"Sir, looks like we've got several potential enemy squirters moving from a house into the field across the street about 150 meters north of your location," said one of the gunship techs.

"Roger that," Jason replied. He quickly called the TOC and relayed what the pilot had told him. Standard operating procedure is typically to make pursuit, so Jason gathered a small team of SEALs, Iraqi counterparts, and their interpreter and moved quickly down the road toward the last known position of the enemy. As they moved to the edge of the field the gunship continued to relay the enemy positions in the thick brush.

"Can you tell if they have weapons?" Jason asked the gunship. "No, sir." Jason called for the team to spread out into a skirmish line, each man about ten meters apart. In a conversation I later had with Jason about this very moment he told me that his Spidey sense was tingling big time. Something just didn't seem right. And if you've ever pursued enemy fighters through extremely thick brush at nighttime, you know that night vision goggles are about as worthless as chicken shit on a pump handle (just some good old Texas slang for you).

Jason requested everyone switch to another frequency so they could communicate with each other while he maintained additional comms with the gunship. But not everyone heard it, so the right and left flak teams ended up on different frequencies. So, when Jason ordered them to push toward the northeast part of the field, the left flank team continued toward the northwest creating a massive gap. Now with almost zero visibility and no solid updates from the gunship, Jason ordered his team to take a knee and wait. A minute later his interpreter approached him and mentioned that the left flank team was no longer there. Shit. They were still on the other frequency and hadn't heard the call.

Jason and his team moved from their position and continued to push toward the northeast edge of the field. The thick brush soon opened to a clearing, a flat dirt lot between the field and adjacent road about fifty meters to the east. As they broke into the clearing Jason's corpsman stepped right on top of a hidden enemy fighter. The fighter tried to roll over but the SEAL delivered a three-round burst to his chest. A firefight immediately ensued—the corpsman taking a round in the leg. Jason called out to the left flank team. "I think that decision really fucked us," he later told me.

All of a sudden, they took a violent barrage of heavy machine gun fire from a barricaded enemy position only twenty meters away. They had walked right into an ambush. Jason took a large caliber round through the elbow and was stitched across the body armor and helmet, his left NVG tube blown clear off. Jason hit the ground, his left forearm dangling by a thread. His other teammates were now behind the only cover in the open area, a tractor tire. Jason was between them and the enemy position with a firefight raging inches above his head. He knew he had to get out of the kill zone to the cover position. Rounds were cracking all around him. He got up and began running. A machine gun round hit him right in front of his right ear and blew out the right side of his face. Down he went. His teammates witnessed what had happened and assumed the worst. They fought on. Jason's team leader and Joint Terminal Attack Controller (JTAC) hopped on the radio and pleaded with the gunship to *drop ordnance danger close.* "Negative. We'll kill you if we drop," they replied.

Alive but unconscious, Jason laid face down in the dirt with a pool of blood quickly expanding beneath him. When he came to, bullets were still flying. He knew he didn't have long to live. He called out to his teammates, shocking them that he was alive. "Give me a headcount! How long until the medevac?" he yelled. "I'm on it, bro, stand by!" the team leader called back.

After reminding them again they could be killed, a gunship crew member requested the SEAL's JTAC number and confirmed the drop. About a minute later, the enemy position was destroyed by heavy ordnance from the gunship. The machine gun fire stopped immediately. Jason's teammates ran to his position and began dragging him as the medevac helo landed thirty meters away. The pain was unbearable, so Jason found his feet and walked unaccompanied the rest of the way. "All I remember is looking down and seeing what seemed like gallons of blood streaming onto my boots as I walked," he told me.

Jason soon found out that he had been shot seven times in the face, chest, and arms. The most devastating round had entered through the right side of his head and exited through his nose— or where his nose used to be. His left elbow had been thoroughly shattered and his forearm was attached only by flesh and tendons.

Jason arrived at the National Naval Medical Center in Bethesda, Maryland, on September 16, 2007. Over the next five years, he endured thirty-seven surgeries and required twelve hundred stitches, two hundred staples, fifteen skin grafts, and one tracheotomy. He lost his sense of smell and has a limited range of motion in his left arm.

While Jason was recovering, he had many visitors, including teammates, family, and friends. But he quickly became frustrated by all the sorrow and tears, so he hung a sign on his hospital door. The bright orange poster read:

> Attention to all who enter here. If you are coming into this room with sorrow or to feel sorry for my wounds, go elsewhere. The wounds I received I got in a job I love, doing it for people I love, supporting the freedom of a country I deeply love. I am incredibly tough and will make a full recovery. What is full? That is the absolute utmost physically my body has the ability to recover. Then I will push that about 20 percent further through sheer mental tenacity. This room you are about to enter is a room of fun, optimism, and intense rapid regrowth. If you are not prepared for that, go elsewhere.
>
> **—The Management**

The sign attracted the attention of then-President George W. Bush, whom Jason later had the chance to meet in the Oval Office. The sign now hangs in the wounded ward of Walter Reed National Military Medical Center.

The doctors provided a laundry list of things Jason would never be able to do again. In public, almost everyone assumed he had been in a terrible car accident or motorcycle crash—nobody ever asked if it had been through military service. He later had a T-shirt made that read: "Stop staring. I got shot by a machine gun. It would have killed you." Jason, and many others with similar stories, live the SEAL Ethos every day. They are still in the fight. No regrets.

Inspired by that? No shit. Me too. Feel kind of stupid because you just screamed a flurry of expletives after stepping on a Lego? Jason has made far more than a full recovery. He fully recovered physically, is in a better state of mind than ever, is happily married with children, and coaches individuals and organizations on his "Overcome" philosophy of resilience and leadership. He's a successful entrepreneur, world-renowned motivational speaker, and two-time best-selling author of *The Trident* and *Overcome*. He's grateful, kind, and still gives to causes greater than himself. Basically, he's a total badass. Not too shabby. The point is that anyone (with the right amount of resolve) can embrace this warrior mindset and overcome seemingly insurmountable odds despite getting dealt some shitty cards. How we view and respond to adversity is a choice.

✪

In 2001, Glenn E. Mangurian suffered an unprovoked disc rupture that left him paralyzed from the waist down. He contends that a traumatic event can cause one to rethink their life, beliefs, and moral convictions. In his *Harvard Business Review* article "Realizing What You're Made Of," he shares six pillars for gaining wisdom through adversity:

1. You can't know what will happen until tomorrow—and it's better that way.
2. You can't control what happens, just how you respond.
3. Adversity distorts reality but crystallizes the truth.
4. Loss amplifies the value of what remains.
5. It's easier to create new dreams than cling to broken ones.
6. Your happiness is more important than righting injustices.

Building resilience—which we will dive deep into in the coming chapters—starts with embracing the suck. Moving from causal thinking and analysis paralysis to action-oriented execution. Moving past the "Why me, why now?" mindset to finding a new path; asking, "What have I gained from this, and how can I use that as fuel for my journey?"

Mental Model

The Five-Step Root Cause Analysis

How often do we spend way too much of our valuable and very limited time dwelling on why awful things happen to us or our loved ones as opposed to finding the root cause (if there is one worth defining) and taking action to move forward? Usually way too much time. Causal thinking and analysis paralysis can keep us locked in our tiny box of mediocrity, content to eat Ritz crackers and watch daytime TV, impairing our ability to learn from bad experiences and take fucking action. Causal reasoning is the process of identifying causality, the relationship between a cause and its effect. The study of causality extends from ancient philosophy to contemporary neuropsychology, but let's keep it simple: I'm basically talking about dwelling on the past. We should *learn* from it, but not *dwell* on it.

On the battlefield, analysis paralysis can literally get you killed. In the moment, you don't have time to ponder a mistake or mourn a fallen teammate who's bleeding out fifteen feet away. When you get pinned down by enemy fire and have to choose between three bad options, you still have to choose. When your platoon commander gets shot in the face, you still have to win the gunfight before you can render any significant aid. Otherwise, more casualties pile up. It sucks, but that's the reality of war.

On your path to embracing the suck and living an extraordinary life, you will be dealt some bad cards. Obstacles crop up in the most untimely manner, be they an enemy ambush, a global pandemic, a citywide riot, or a horrible medical prognosis. So what? Control what you can and deprioritize what you can't.

There is a big difference between being trapped in causal reflection and applying lessons learned to take action. When we can transform our minds toward action-oriented thinking by accepting life's sick little jokes and learning what we can along the way, awesomeness and winning are sure to follow. Just remember, *winning* never comes without *adversity*. They are joined at the hip.

If it doesn't involve at least a little bit of pain, adversity, or challenge, it's not worth doing.

You have goals for your life, right? If not, you're a loser and this book won't help you. But assuming you do, please keep reading. When have you ever achieved anything truly fulfilling without some challenges along the way? Never. If you have, the goal wasn't that great in the first place. Sorry, I'm just saying. Maybe it's starting a business or family, getting into a great school, developing your skills at a sport you love, growing a vegetable garden, raising your children, mastering the art of walking on stilts, or being elected president. Whatever the goal, there are always obstacles and bad cards to contend with along the way. Businesses fail. Families fall apart. Schools deny applications. Coaches pick other players. Gardens get ransacked by teams of hungry special ops vermin that attack in the night (those fuckers ruined our garden, by the way). Children become teenagers. Only a weirdo would feel the need to master the art of stilt-walking. And not just anyone can become president—although I'm starting to think that's not the case anymore. But let's not go down the politics rabbit hole right now.

You can't always control what the Wheel of Misfortune has in store for you or when and where you'll get hit with enemy fire, but you *can* control what you learn from these experiences and how you fight back. You can wallow in misery or tell tragedy to go fuck itself with the mindset David Goggins explains in his book *Can't Hurt Me*. You can drop heavy ordnance on that enemy position, get up, dust yourself off, and live to fight another day. When obstacles strike (and they will), you need to identify the root cause, apply lessons learned, and move on with life.

How? By using the Embrace the Suck Five-Step Root Cause Analysis mental model.

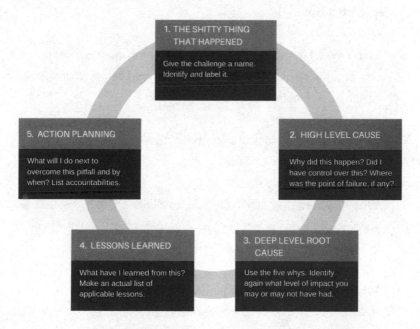

1. THE SHITTY THING THAT HAPPENED
Give the challenge a name. Identify and label it.

2. HIGH LEVEL CAUSE
Why did this happen? Did I have control over this? Where was the point of failure, if any?

3. DEEP LEVEL ROOT CAUSE
Use the five whys. Identify again what level of impact you may or may not have had.

4. LESSONS LEARNED
What have I learned from this? Make an actual list of applicable lessons.

5. ACTION PLANNING
What will I do next to overcome this pitfall and by when? List accountabilities.

For example, let's say you lost your job. That's *The Shitty Thing That Happened*. It was unexpected, came out of nowhere with no significant indicators and no lengthy explanation from your manager. Okay, so now you have a name for the problem. Now you ask yourself why you think this happened. Make a list of possibilities both in your control and potentially out of your control. Let's say, hypothetically speaking, that the company is in financial strain due to an unforeseen global pandemic and downsizing your division, while keeping their top performers—you're apparently not one of them. There's your *High Level Cause.*

Okay, why? Move to step three to identify the *Deep Level Root Cause,* only focusing on the aspects in your control—actual or perceived underperformance. Don't dwell on anything beyond your sphere of influence. Ask yourself *why* five times, digging deeper each time.

Why? Well, I guess I could have taken more ownership over my role regardless of the lack of clarity provided by my manager (who's an asshole, by the way).

Why? There was a lack of clarity because it wasn't provided but, most importantly, I didn't ask.

Why? Because I'd been in this role for a year and felt unsafe in shedding light on the fact that I wasn't totally clear about my role or how I contributed to mission success.

Why? I suppose my manager doesn't really foster an environment of psychological safety, but I was also relatively comfortable doing the bare minimum.

Why? The star players who were "all in" had a lot more work to do and were always called upon to take on new projects. I enjoyed leaving at 5:00 p.m. every day to go to yoga. Well damn, now I have no job but plenty of time for yoga (but the studio closed), wallowing in misery, and walking my Shih Tzu in the park by my apartment—which I now can't afford.

Move to step four and make a list of your *Lessons Learned*. Perform your personal after-action review. Ask: what did I do well, what did I not do so well, and what will I change to enhance my performance? Document your findings. With that data, you are now ready for *Action Planning*. Make it specific. And make sure your goals are concise, realistic, and time bound. We'll get into the Embrace the Suck action planning model later, but start with a simple objective statement such as "to never lose another job for underperformance."

But sometimes things aren't so clear cut. Have you ever experienced stress or anxiety but were unsure what was really driving those feelings? Sometimes it's truly as easy as using this simple tool. Interestingly enough, I often find that what I've initially labeled as the *Shitty Thing* isn't even what's causing the stress. When we mislabel what we're worrying about, we are ill-equipped to develop the proper plan of action to alleviate the anxiety. Once properly identified, you can develop a plan of attack that only addresses the elements that are under your control.

By using this model in its simplest form, the process becomes muscle memory. It becomes your natural state of mind when faced with adversity. You continue to build mental calluses and emotional fortitude by executing your action plans. Your personal feedback loops place you in a constant state of course correction and improvement. You bounce back faster each time tragedy strikes. Your perception of adversity and its impact on you and those around you evolves.

Did Jason get shot in the face? You're damn right he did. He was already a great combat leader, and now he's an even stronger person for it. He didn't waste a second crying about it. He walked his bad ass to that medevac helicopter and never looked back. He turned tragedy into a tool for inspiring others. Pretty fucking cool in my opinion.

Great, So What Now?

Well, now you start using this approach. Test yourself. Reflect on how you've reacted in the past when dealt crappy cards and measure how quickly you recovered. Build a baseline to improve upon. How long did it take you to course correct? To shift fire on the battlefield? To call for air support? Be open to learning from others you know who had to become more resilient just to survive tragedy—be it a brain tumor, divorce, car crash, getting fired, losing a small business, being laid off, or taking a little point-blank machine gun fire. How did they get through it? You'd be surprised. Once you open up and start sharing your struggles with others you trust, you'll always find people who have been through much worse. Use that knowledge to gain perspective.

Identify the root causes of your failures, pain, and barriers to happiness, then develop a plan and execute, execute, execute.

Questions to ask yourself:

When I get knocked down, do I get back up quickly or tend to drown in self-pity?

Do I trend initially toward surprise, denial, and anger when given feedback or do I accept it and take action?

What have I learned from the adversity I have experienced in my life? Did I apply that to make positive changes? If so, have I been consistent in applying those changes?

Do I spend too much time analyzing what's beyond my control or find the silver lining and move forward?

How am I going to hold myself accountable to using the Five-Step Root Cause Analysis mental model?

3

OH, AND MAYBE YOUR VALUES ARE ALL WRONG

Values are like fingerprints. Nobody's are the same but you leave them all over everything you do.

—ELVIS PRESLEY

Why do horrible and unjust things happen to good people? Why are kind people inflicted with terminal illnesses while evil and selfish people seem to breeze through life without a scratch? Why do people of great principle die young before having the opportunity to get married, have children, or leave their mark on the world? If you are a person of faith (whatever faith that may be), you most likely believe there is a greater plan for each of us—a plan we will never fully understand and that may only come to fruition when we stay true to our values. (Assuming those values don't suck, of course.) Core values are the fundamental beliefs of a person or organization. These guiding principles ideally dictate behavior and can help us understand the difference between right and wrong. When clearly defined, they provide a beacon that keeps us on the path to an extraordinary life.

BUD/S Class 235 Hell Week
March 2001, Coronado, California
10:05 P.M.

By Wednesday night, there were only about forty students remaining in class 235. We were running on fumes, delirious from sleep deprivation and the sensory overload that comes with nonstop pain. But we were starting to see the light at the end of the torture tunnel. Some in our class had been rolled back for injuries and would pick up with the next class once they'd healed. But most had decided this life wasn't for them. Soon after each man succumbed to the suffering and could embrace no more suck, they went to the infamous courtyard—called "The Grinder"— and rang the bell that hangs there, then placed their green helmet in line with the others.

It had been raining for three days. I had no skin left on my knees, between my legs, around my waist, in my armpits, or on the top of my head. My nipples were bloody nubs. I was covered in blisters. The severe sting of the saltwater on the open wounds was a nice touch as well. Oh, and my elbow was, of course, still fractured. One of my buddies who was in my crew actually had two broken shins—but he suffered through the extreme pain in silence so he could finish Hell Week.

We stood at attention on the pool deck awaiting further instructions for our next evolution—the caterpillar swim. I wish it were as cute as it sounds—like an activity at a little kid's birthday party—but that's unfortunately not the case. Our class leader, John, was hunched over on the stairs gasping for air. He was suffering from severe pneumonia and his lung air sacs, alveoli, were filling with fluid as each hour passed. He'd been in med checks all week, but still led the class like the passionate professional he was. But John now looked worse than any of us. The instructors asked him if he could continue and, of course, he said he could. But by the look of his physical state, I feared he wouldn't make it much further.

They ordered the lot of us to get in the pool with our boat crews. We were fully clothed. The caterpillar swim is a race against the other crews. The students in each boat crew are swimming on their backs, legs wrapped around the waist of the man in front of him, using only their arms for propulsion. The evolution is very difficult when you're fresh, so imagine the challenge it posed four days into Hell Week. My crew was halfway down the length of the Olympic-size swimming pool when two instructors dove into the water. Another instructor with a megaphone told us to exit the pool and sit along the fence facing the opposite direction with our heads down. John's body had gone limp and sunk to the bottom of the nine-foot section like he was wearing cement boots. We heard the panic in their voices as they tried to revive him. They then quickly loaded him in the ambulance that was on standby. The class was told to run back across the street to the training center and wait in the classroom.

A few hours later, we still waited, exhausted and confused. All of a sudden, the door opened and the commanding officer of BUD/S walked in and headed straight to the front of the room. He wasted no time.

"Mr. Skop is dead. Mr. Porado, you're the new class leader," he said, looking at the officer who was second in command.

He paused to let the news sink in. It was like we'd been kicked in the gut, already fragile from injury, illness, and sleep deprivation. Tears streamed down cheeks, flowing from eyes bearing a thousand-yard stare. "Gents, get used to this. This will most likely be the first of many brothers you'll lose. And unfortunately, we have to secure Hell Week now. You guys are done." Then he left the room like it was just another fucked-up day at the office.

A wave of guilt hit me as soon as I felt the relief of hearing those words. We were done. We'd finished Hell Week—the toughest week of military training known to man. But we were done because John was dead. I struggled to comprehend the meaning of it all, having never lost anyone close to me before. The commanding officer's words unintentionally foreshadowed the events to come. The 9/11 attacks occurred a few months later, and I can't even recall how many SEAL funerals I've been to since. Too many.

John was a man who lived by a set of solid core values. He was a well-respected leader who didn't deserve to die. It goes to show that life can be very short—why waste a second of it living misguided by a poor set of values?

As they say, the show must go on. The following week, training resumed. Since our Hell Week had been secured a day early, the instructors needed to exact their vengeance. Normally, the week after Hell Week is called "walk week." Your body is so broken they don't demand the usual sixty miles per week of running. You're allowed to walk. But there was no walk week for class 235. We got beat harder and more viciously than ever. It was punishment. Bad cards being dealt each day. But we didn't give a shit. We had a mission to complete. The pain of losing John was the fuel needed for our journey.

✪

As I previously mentioned, the Naval Special Warfare community has invested millions of dollars in research trying to identify
the cognitive, physical, and emotional attributes of the students
who are most likely to graduate. The most interesting data points
are centered on the difficult to measure but important aspects of
shared values, emotional maturity, and a deep passion to serve.
Feeling connected to the mission carries guys through the most
painful times. They have a vision that *must* be fulfilled, a goal so
important that nothing will stand in their way. They have core values that mesh well with the SEAL community.

Every decision we make is either a conscious or unconscious
attempt to satisfy our needs. Even in SEAL training. Over time,
humans have developed six ways of making decisions—instincts,
subconscious beliefs, conscious beliefs, intuition, inspiration,
and values.

Values are an integral part of life and they play an important
role in the way our lives unfold. They are, of course, highly personal and can vary significantly from person to person. It's important that you know what your values are, so you can make the best
possible decisions for executing your personal *mission plan*.

It's important to ask ourselves the following questions:

What do I value most in life?

What is my ultimate purpose? My why?

What is my plan for fulfilling that purpose?

If we can't answer these questions with conviction, it becomes
very challenging to align our decisions, activities, and behaviors
with achieving our goals. Our values will be tested many times on
the battlefield of life, and our experiences can shape those values,

for better or worse. And sometimes, even when we have clearly defined those values, we lose sight of them.

But what if one day you realize—or are told—that you have shitty values? And maybe those values are leading you in the wrong direction? Or possibly driving you to pursue goals for all the wrong reasons? Consider a guy I used to know, let's call him Jeff. He was an intelligent, eager young entrepreneur who'd found some relative success with his first couple of ventures after grad school. He was driven by money and the notion of prominence, but also suffered from a solid case of "only child" syndrome. He was entitled and selfish. All his personal and professional goals revolved around acquiring more things. More money. A bigger house. A Ferrari by a certain age. The list goes on and on.

One day, Jeff was complaining to me about his marriage—his "bipolar" wife, their constant fighting. He was bitching about how she was always yelling at him for not helping with the baby, taking out the trash, or fixing the broken kitchen drawer. I listened, pondering his point of view but trying to understand hers as well. I knew the guy really well, so I asked him how he planned to address these common but unavoidable realities of a marriage partnership. His prizewinning response was that he'd prioritize his wife and kid once his start-up reached a certain revenue goal. Yep! A certain revenue goal. As if it was part of his business plan. *When revenue hits X, I will fix Y.* You can't make this up.

After a brief pause, I responded, "Okay, sooooo you're telling me you will prioritize your family—*your family*—only after your company reaches X revenue, which potentially, or most likely, has an unforeseen timeline?" Of course, what I was really thinking was, *They won't be around by the time that event occurs, if it ever does.* "Yes, that's exactly what I'm saying. I just can't focus on that right now," he confirmed. His firm conviction made it even more shocking.

His values seemed to be . . . what's the phrase I'm looking for . . . total shit! Not to mention I knew he was using "business trips" as a reason to engage in extreme debauchery and play poker all night. He's another reason I don't care for poker, by the way. Did his wife have anger issues? Ya think?!

You see, Jeff had perfectly normal aspirations for a young entrepreneur: growth, monetary reward, building something great, providing jobs, and creating shareholder value. But he was also doing it at the expense of others and based on a totally mis-guided set of values. Not long after that conversation, his wife left him and they entered an emotionally (and financially) costly divorce process. He soared to new heights of pill-popping, anxi-ety rendering him incapable of properly leading his business to the next level. It never even came close to reaching that revenue target, and his business was sold for its debt years later. He learned valuable lessons from these experiences and went on to do great things. But I assume he always asks, "What if?"

If our values don't align with what we want out of life—I mean, of course, the things that really matter—then we face far greater challenges than when they do. Sometimes our perspective is skewed. We chase the wrong dreams and faulty aspirations that leave us empty, void unfulfilled.

One of my favorite poems is all about living a life of value, knowing your core values, and living by them every day. The poem is titled "Death Song," and it was written by Tecumseh. Tecumseh was a Native American Shawnee warrior and chief, who became the primary leader of a large, multi-tribal confederacy in the early nineteenth century. Born in the Ohio Country (present-day Ohio), and growing up during the American Revolutionary War and the Northwest Indian War, Tecumseh was exposed to warfare and envisioned the establishment of an independent Native American nation east of the Mississippi River under British protection. Tecumseh was among the most celebrated Native American leaders in history and was known as a strong and eloquent orator who promoted tribal unity. He was also ambitious, willing to take risks, and make significant sacrifices to repel the Americans from Native American lands in the Old Northwest Territory.

The poem is widely shared in the Naval Special Warfare community, and in many ways captures our values and how we approach life and work.

So live your life that the fear of death can never enter your heart. Trouble no one about their religion; respect others in their view, and demand that they respect yours. Love your life, perfect your life, and beautify all things in your life. Seek to make your life long and its purpose in the service of your people. Prepare a noble death song for the day when you go over the great divide.

Always give a word or a sign of salute when meeting or passing a friend, even a stranger, when in a lonely place. Show respect to all people and grovel to none.

When you arise in the morning give thanks for the light, your strength, the food, and for the joy of living. If you see no reason for giving

*thanks, the fault lies only in yourself. Abuse no
one and no thing, for abuse turns the wise ones
to fools and robs the spirit of its vision.*

*When it comes your time to die, be not like
those whose hearts are filled with the fear of
death, so that when their time comes they weep
and pray for a little more time to live their lives
over again in a different way. Sing your death
song and die like a hero going home.*

The last paragraph has the most impact on me. It's about living with the end in mind—your personal exit strategy, if you will. It challenges you to define what winning looks like and work backward from there, rather than leaving your list of regrets to chance. Personal transformation in the embrace the suck journey often involves values analysis before you can start getting comfortable being uncomfortable, and auditing our moral convictions so they are authentic and in line with what we want out of this short life.

James Clear, American author, entrepreneur, and world-famous photographer, says, "Making better choices is often a matter of choosing better constraints. By limiting your options to those that fit your values, you are taking an important step to ensuring that your behavior matches your beliefs. Plus, constraints will boost your creativity. Know your principles and you can choose your methods." Essentially, any action or choice should clearly fit within your value lane markers. Deviation outside those markers typically ends in tragedy. Again, that assumes your values don't suck. You need to ask yourself what you are willing to do to live by those values and, even more importantly, what you are unwilling to do to avoid deviation.

John Skop was a man of great values and solid moral conviction. He had been an intel officer at SEAL Team One prior to joining BUD/S class 235. His values drove his decision to take his service to this great nation to the next level. He cared so deeply about becoming a SEAL and giving to a cause greater than himself that he was willing to risk it all in chasing that dream. His paddle is a constant reminder to me of the importance of living a values-driven life.

Mental Model

The Personal Values Manifesto

Since 9/11, the NSW community has constantly applied lessons learned on the battlefield to adjust its conflict strategies and tactics. Our ethos is essentially the culture statement that guides who we are and why we exist. It defines our values. By 2005, we had been operating in volatile and uncertain environments for four years, but we'd never taken the time to clearly articulate who we are as a team, a community. What do we stand for? What's our true purpose? Why do we exist? What do we expect of ourselves and each other? What foundation exists from which we make our decisions? What values not only define us, but who we want to bring into our crazy little world? So, in 2005, a leadership off-site event was scheduled. Sounds very corporate, right? The goal was to create the NSW credo. And thus, the Navy SEAL Ethos was born:

> In times of war or uncertainty there is a special breed of warrior ready to answer our nation's call. A common man with an

uncommon desire to succeed. Forged by adversity, he stands alongside America's finest special operations forces to serve his country, the American people, and protect their way of life. I am that man.

My Trident is a symbol of honor and heritage. Bestowed upon me by the heroes that have gone before, it embodies the trust of those I have sworn to protect. By wearing the Trident I accept the responsibility of my chosen profession and way of life. It is a privilege that I must earn every day. My loyalty to country and team is beyond reproach. I humbly serve as a guardian to my fellow Americans always ready to defend those who are unable to defend themselves. I do not advertise the nature of my work, nor seek recognition for my actions. I voluntarily accept the inherent hazards of my profession, placing the welfare and security of others before my own. I serve with honor on and off the battlefield. The ability to control my emotions and my actions, regardless of circumstances, sets me apart from other men. Uncompromising integrity is my standard. My character and honor are steadfast. My word is my bond.

We expect to lead and be led. In the absence of orders, I will take charge, lead my teammates, and accomplish the mission. I lead by example in all situations. I will never quit. I persevere and thrive on adversity. My Nation expects me to be physically harder and mentally stronger than my enemies. If knocked down, I will get back up, every time. I will draw on every remaining ounce of strength to protect my teammates and to accomplish our mission. I am never out of the fight.

We demand discipline. We expect innovation. The lives of my teammates and the success of our mission depends on me— my technical skill, tactical proficiency, and attention to detail. My training is never complete.

We train for war and fight to win. I stand ready to bring the full spectrum of combat power to bear in order to achieve my mission and the goals established by my country. The execution of my duties will be swift and violent when required yet guided by the very principles that I serve to defend. Brave men have fought and died building the proud tradition and feared reputation that I am bound to uphold. In the worst of conditions, the legacy of my teammates steadies my resolve and silently guides my every deed.

I will not fail.

Let's break this down. In the first paragraph we define who we are and state the fact that "I am that man." If I couldn't have authentically believed that *I am that man* the day I began BUD/S, I would have had no business being there. The most powerful statement related to values, however, is: "The execution of my duties will be swift and violent when required *yet guided by the very principles that I serve to defend*." Regardless of the goal, when we sacrifice our values in an effort to achieve that goal, all is lost. Earning the Trident pin is truly a privilege bestowed on us by the heroes who have gone before—a privilege we earn, not once, but every single day.

Have you ever taken the time to write down your values? You've probably thought about them or even talked about what matters most to you, but have you actually documented your core beliefs and values? If you have, did you also apply the behaviors you expect from yourself and others, as well as specific ways to hold yourself accountable? If special operations units, winning sports teams, and high-performing business organizations do it, why shouldn't we do it for ourselves?

So if you haven't, let's do that now using the Personal Values Manifesto mental model—which consists of clearly defined core values, supporting behaviors, and accountability mechanisms.

STEP ONE: Get off your ass and go get a pad of Post-it Notes. Yes, now, please. Find a quiet place void of toddlers, coworkers, lawn mowers, clowns, and terrorists. Grab yourself a good pen with plenty of ink. Start by writing one core value on each Post-it. For example, faith, integrity, wellness, family, etc. Remember, they must be meaningful to you. Authentic. Not values you think others would like to see you have. There can be an aspirational element to each—something to aspire to improve or live by more closely—but they have to be real. Write down as many as you can think of. Don't worry about themes or redundancy. We'll get to categorization later.

STEP TWO: Okay, now you have a pile of pink Post-it Notes with very inspiring and thought-provoking shit on them. You're saying to yourself, *Man, I value lots of stuff, this is great.* If you only have one or two Post-its, you're a lost cause. Just kidding—keep at it, then come back to this step. Now categorize them into themes as best you can. Group them into piles, stick them on the window, the mirror, a white board, whatever works best. You will dive deeper when you detail the supporting behaviors and accountability mechanisms in the next step, but for now, narrow it down to between four and six core values.

STEP THREE: Now you are ready to list Supporting Behaviors for each core value. For example, if integrity is a value, what does that mean to you specifically? What behavioral norms are you going to live by that support your value of integrity? What lengths are you willing to go to and what are you absolutely unwilling to do in order to live by that value? If wellness is a value, what are you going to do every day to embody that value? Get up at a specific time for exercise? Set time-bound goals? Design a new dietary plan? And no, I'm not talking about New Year's resolutions—that shit's for losers. These are things you're going to do consistently year-round, day in and day out. A lifestyle. Make a short and concise list of two or three supporting behaviors for each value.

STEP FOUR: Great, you've listed your supporting behaviors. Now what? How will you hold yourself accountable? Be as specific as possible. List at least one accountability mechanism for each behavior. For example, if a supporting behavior is to make time for daily exercise, your accountability mechanism might be to set an alarm for 5:00 a.m. each day, or 4:30 a.m. if you're super hardcore. You can also have others hold you accountable; tell everyone you're doing this. When you stray, which you will, define how you will get back on track.

STEP FIVE: Put it all on paper. Print it out. Laminate it. Keep it on your desk. Tattoo it on the back of your eyelids. Build an app that sends you reminders—but please throw me a bone when you sell it for beaucoup bucks!

When our consulting firm takes clients through this exercise, the outcome is called a Team Charter, and it defines the values, behaviors, and accountabilities that are used for everything from talent acquisition and onboarding to training, performance management systems, and decision-making. And again, if high-performance teams use this model, why shouldn't we use it for ourselves or our families?

Great, So What Now?

Don't be like Jeff. Be like John. John was called over the great divide as a young man, but he lived each day leading up to that fateful night in Hell Week by a set of authentic core values. That's why he was loved. That's why he is deeply missed.

If you take the time to make it real, your Personal Values Manifesto will not only guide you to new heights, it will help you avoid the many pitfalls of temptation. So get after it.

Questions to ask yourself:

When was the last time I audited my value system?

Do I make decisions based on a specific moral code?
If I have one, how often do I stray from it?

How has adversity shaped my values? How have they transformed?

Am I being honest with myself about how my priorities align with my values?

Am I willing to use this tool and apply it every day?

4

TAMING TEMPTATION TIGER

I can resist anything except temptation.

—OSCAR WILDE, *LADY WINDERMERE'S FAN*

Imagine you're standing on a cliff's edge, surrounded by thick green jungle foliage for as far as the eye can see. Colorful birds chirping in the distance. On the other side of the vast precipice is Glory Town, where your life goals, ambitions, and delusions of grandeur reside. Unbeknownst to you, the bottom of the ravine is where Temptation Tiger lives. You've heard the rumors of his immense power. Legend has it that many have ventured into his lair, never to return.

As you gaze longingly at the magical glow of Glory Town (where your dreams will come true with no real effort or adversity) contemplating a way across the ravine, you notice some movement below. Temptation Tiger casually strolls out of a dark cave. He has a Grey Goose martini in one paw, a perfectly rolled joint in the other paw, and a smokin' hot lady tiger on each arm. His fur is glossy and well-maintained. His teeth are white as polished ivory. He's wearing a red silk smoking jacket and a purple paisley ascot tie. You think to yourself, *Huh, he doesn't seem so bad. He's clearly legit!*

He looks up, catches your gaze, and says, "Come on down, we're having a little get-together tonight. You should join us— the more the merrier! Plenty of booze, cannabis, heavy hors d'oeuvres, and pretty girls. Gonna get a poker game going later too. Oh, and all the other players suck, so don't worry. Your chances of winning big are high!"

Well, I do enjoy a good game of poker, you think. *I'm not great, but good enough. The extra cash would definitely come in handy for the rest of my journey. And I could really use a drink—it's hot as hell out here. And who doesn't like shrimp pot stickers and pretty lady tigers? I'll just swing by for a bit and then head toward Glory Town later.*

With a slight bit of trepidation (and a small voice in the back of your mind questioning your judgment), you find a nice thick vine and begin to shimmy down the cliff face. Once you reach the bottom, Temptation Tiger strolls over with outstretched arms and a toothy grin and gives you a warm hug. His furry embrace instantly makes you feel safe. The voice of reason in your head vanishes and you're confident in your decision. *Glory Town can wait a little while. Let's get this party started!* Out of nowhere, the music starts bumping and fireworks burst into the fading light of dusk.

Remember how things turned out for Jeff? The next morning you wake up with a raging headache, dizzy and still a bit stoned, with no money and no lady tigers. Oh, and there seems to be no rope ladder to climb up the other side toward your *real* dreams. Your headache suddenly gets worse. Glory Town now seems out of reach. Anxiety and regret set in. All is lost. You realize that you allowed temptation to lure you down the wrong path, outside of the healthy constraints of your values. Can you recover from this? Most likely. Was this avoidable? Absolutely.

✪

Sometimes, Temptation Tiger really bites us in the ass. Literally. Take Vladimir Markov. He was a selfish and misguided poacher (and ironically also a beekeeper) who met a grisly end in the winter of 1997 after he shot and wounded a tiger, then stole part of the tiger's kill.

The most biodiverse region in all of Russia lies on a chunk of land sandwiched between China and the Pacific Ocean. There, in Russia's Far East, subarctic animals—such as caribou and wolves—mingle with tigers and other species of the subtropics. It was very nearly a perfect habitat for the tigers until humans showed up.

The tigers that populate this region are commonly called Siberian tigers, but they are more accurately known as the Amur tiger. Imagine a creature that has the agility and appetite of a cat and the mass of an industrial refrigerator. The Amur tiger can weigh over 500 pounds and can be more than 10 feet long, nose to tail. These majestic tigers can jump as far as 25 feet; vertically, they can jump over a basketball hoop. They are obviously not to be trifled with.

Nevertheless, one day Markov and his shitty values came across a tiger who was gnawing on a fresh kill. Driven by greed, temptation, and the accumulation of relatively insignificant wealth, Markov thought to himself, *Perfect! Two birds with one stone. A kill to eat and a tiger to sell on the black market.* Markov took aim and shot the tiger, but he only wounded him. The tiger ran off into the woods, hungry and really pissed off. So, while licking his wounds, the tiger developed his plan for taking revenge: a good old-fashioned Navy SEAL–style ambush.

A couple days later, the injured tiger hunted down Markov in a way that appears to be chillingly premeditated. The tiger staked out Markov's cabin, systematically destroyed anything that had Markov's scent on it, then waited by the front door for Markov to come home. Martini in one hand, joint in the other. Instead of a smoking jacket, he was cloaked in rage. When Markov returned to the cabin, the tiger flicked the joint to the ground, gently set his drink on the table, then swiftly and violently took his vengeance. He dragged Markov into the forest, killed, and ate him. All that remained of the beekeeper were stumps of bone sticking out of his boots, a bloodied shirt with an arm still inside, a severed hand, a faceless head, and a gnawed femur.

The moral of the story? Only shoot things that deserve to be shot. Don't steal. Don't poach. And don't let temptation lead you to make poor decisions, or you too may end up just like Markov, bloody stumps and all.

✪

Crested Butte, Colorado
May 2000

Crunch ... crunch ... crunch. My Oakley hiking boots penetrated the freshly fallen snow with every labored step. The sun had just begun climbing slowly over the horizon, but the KÜHL pants and Under Armour T-shirt I was wearing were already dampening with sweat. My chest was heaving with each labored breath in the thin Colorado air at eleven thousand feet altitude. My twin brother and college buddy followed closely behind me, our day packs full of climbing gear, cans of tuna, peanut butter crackers, and plenty of water—two full Nalgene bottles each. A storm would be setting in later that day, and we needed to make the peak by early afternoon so we wouldn't miss our turnaround window. This was the third time in a week we'd made this steep ascent; it was part of our ridiculous training regimen. My buddy Matt from Southern Methodist University and I had been living in Crested Butte for a couple months, training for ten to twelve hours a day for the Navy SEAL selection program. I was in the best condition of my life—at least up to that point.

But let's back up a bit. I grew up in Dallas, Texas, in an upper middle-class family with my mom, dad, twin brother, and a yellow lab named Jenny. We lived in a white ranch-style house on Prestonshire Lane. My brother and I both attended St. Michael's for elementary school, followed by the Episcopal School of Dallas (ESD) for middle school. Coincidentally, one of my BUD/S classmates, SEAL Team Five teammates, and now dear friend was at ESD at the same time—but I wouldn't find that out until years later. My dad was a successful commercial real estate pro and Mom was a speech pathologist. She also did a lot of volunteer work through the Junior League in her spare time. Life was pretty good, with no real adversity to speak of.

We attended Jesuit College Preparatory School of Dallas for high school. We initially weren't thrilled about leaving ESD, but we weren't given a choice. It turned out to be an amazing experience. I joined the swim team my freshman year. Apparently, the team needed someone with a strong backstroke. I was a freestyle guy myself and I hated backstroke, but I was the new guy, so guess who got to embrace that suck? Gleeson did. I know, I know. Get some *real* problems, right?!

Anyway, high school was going pretty well. Around the latter part of sophomore year, I reconnected with my best friend from elementary school. He was attending the public school that I would have gone to had I not been in private school, Hillcrest High School. Unfortunately, Temptation Tiger had already started sinking his claws into this young man's cerebral cortex. He'd skip school, drink, and hang out with the other "cool" kids. He was known as a tough guy, good fighter, and a lady's man. He was a bad boy and I wanted a piece of that action. We started hanging out again. This was a very different crowd, socially speaking. But there seemed to be a pattern. My Jesuit buddies—when not distracted by sports, academics, and charity work—liked to drink beer, listen to country music, and engage in the occasional brawl. If that ain't Texas, I don't know what is. This other crew liked to drink, listen to rap music, and fight. So essentially, there was temptation all around, and I made no real effort to avoid the tiger's warm embrace.

I had a fire burning deep inside my soul. It wasn't driven by childhood abuse or poverty; no this was something else. I wanted to experience things outside of my sheltered existence, the good, bad, and ugly. So I did. One day, I challenged one of Dallas's biggest high school bullies to fight me for retribution from another incident. He was two years older, a football player, twice my size, and an asshole to boot. He was always picking on people, like Biff Tannen from *Back to the Future*. Meanwhile, I was a swimmer who played drums in the jazz band. I'm not totally sure why I did it. I assume I wanted to prove something to myself in an immature, misguided high school kind of way. And, of course, I wanted to reap the glory and respect from my soon-to-be victory.

Let's just say it didn't turn out well. Like something out of a movie, we met at a pre-designated time next to a dumpster behind a pizza restaurant. Crowds began to swarm—my camp and his. He pulled up in a blue Ford Mustang, got out, and left the loud rumbling engine running. I assumed we'd talk some more shit and feel each other out before getting our hands dirty. We'd shove each other a bit, then people would jump in to break it up. Easy day. I'd check the box and be a hero. Glory and accolades would soon follow.

Nope. He walked right up and knocked me the fuck out—or so I'm told. With my limp jazz-drumming body on the ground, he then kicked me in the head to finish me off. He may have spit on me too. Not sure.

I regained consciousness in the car. My bad-influence-of-a-friend was driving me home. Yes, that's correct. My very own Temptation Tiger. "What happened? Did I win?" I slurred in my bloody haze. "Haha, hell no. You got your ass kicked, stupid!" he laughed. In his defense, he was actually concerned. I flipped the passenger side mirror down and went into panic mode. "My parents are going to kill me!" I groaned.

So first, I wasn't supposed to be hanging out with him. My parents had forbidden it after a high-speed car chase involving Dallas's finest, but that's a story for another time. Anyway, I clearly had a broken nose and the areas around both eyes were starting to turn that fun purple-yellow color. My jaw was very sore, and I was spitting gravel into my hand. *Damn. That's not gravel. Those are teeth. I am sooooooo screwed. There is no way to hide this one.*

I walked into the house and my mom saw my face from across the kitchen. "Oh my gosh, what happened?!" she said in a panicky Dallas accent. "I ran into a wall playing football after school,"

I replied sheepishly. Yes, that's all I could come up with. She kind of bought the lie at first, but she was clearly skeptical. When my dad got home and saw me, he suspected what had happened but didn't say anything, probably trying to spare my mom more grief. I saw that idiot years later at a holiday party in Dallas after joining the SEAL Teams. He looked a lot less intimidating.

Luckily, I still graduated from Jesuit with decent grades and began college at Southern Methodist University in August of 1995. I made the rugby team freshman year and fell in love with the sport. There was no more swimming nonsense; it was time to crack some skulls! I became close friends with a guy named Matt from Lubbock, Texas—a fraternity brother a year behind me in school. We started hanging out more and I quickly learned of his dream to become a Navy SEAL. I didn't know much about the SEAL Teams at the time other than the fact that they were invincible gods of war! And, of course, glass-eating, fire-breathing behemoths. I'd read a couple books about SEALs in Vietnam, but that was about it. At that stage, I had no real intention of serving in the military.

I graduated in May of 1999 and took a job as a financial analyst at Trammell Crow Company. Matt was a senior and began training hard for the Navy. I trained with him on nights and weekends, but I had no intention of joining him on this ridiculous journey of "nautical nonsense" (yes, I'm borrowing that phrase from Sponge-Bob SquarePants). Every night when I arrived home from work, I would quickly change, throw some swim fins and goggles in a backpack, and run four miles to the SMU natatorium from my downtown apartment. Matt and I would swim for about an hour, mostly freestyle and combat sidestroke, the stroke of choice for the entrance PT test. After busting out some push-ups, sit-ups, and pull-ups on the pool deck, I would run four miles home, make a late dinner, go to bed, then do it all again the next day. On the weekends we would run one or two laps around White Rock Lake—which is a nearly ten-mile loop.

At the time, distance running wasn't my thing. It sucked. But I gradually started loving the pain, and I became addicted to the endorphin high afterward. As a wise SEAL once said, *All you need is a pair of shoes, shorts, and a place to puke.* We signed up for the Dallas White Rock Marathon, which was the first race for both of us. The goal: run the 26.2 miles in under three-and-a-half hours without walking a single step. Maybe that doesn't seem like that big a deal for you runners out there, but back then, believe me, it was. I was too big from having intentionally gained weight for rugby. So, at 6'1" and 220 pounds, I wasn't exactly built for distance. I needed to transform mind and body.

Before and after our workouts, Matt and I had long conversations about the history of the Naval Special Warfare community, the missions, the mindset, everything. We were fascinated. At work, I sat at my desk on the forty-second floor of a downtown high-rise building daydreaming about what it might be like. Matt and I started training harder. I started reading more about the Teams. One day, everything clicked. I felt a call to serve. A need to engage in purposeful suffering. To test myself. To reassess my values. To give to a cause greater than myself.

The next day, I started removing every element of temptation from my life that stood in the path of my new goal; become a SEAL. The tiger had to go. I more or less eliminated my social life—not that it was that great in the first place. I changed my dietary habits and daily routines. I even removed people from my life who were a negative distraction. All my behaviors and accountability mechanisms had to be totally aligned to achieve one goal. My new philosophy: Remove every opportunity for temptation and distraction—any obstacle or competing priority. Maintain total mission focus.

About a month later, I gave my notice to the firm, packed my things, and Matt and I moved to Crested Butte, Colorado, to train at high altitude. It was a place where Temptation Tiger could never find us. We brought long, thick nylon ropes and hung them high in cypress trees to climb daily and build upper body strength. We cut an eight-foot log from a fallen tree to carry with us on trail runs. Using that same log, we performed *log PT*, just like we would in BUD/S. We swam in ice-covered lakes, training our bodies to accept extreme conditions. We ran for miles on mountain trails each day. Climbed tall mountains. Did endless calisthenics. Any punishment we could think of, we did. And we didn't train in REI's finest athletic gear either. Other than the days we did the long mountain ascents, we wore the same uncomfortable battle dress uniforms and boots we would be wearing in BUD/S. After several months, we were ready. We left for Navy boot camp soon after returning home. During boot camp we performed the SEAL PT test—running, swimming, push-ups, pull-ups, sit-ups. The test begins with the 500-meter swim, a mass of bodies sprinting back and forth in the indoor pool. One poor kid almost drowned and had to be pulled from the water. He must have showed up by mistake. At the end of that day, only three of us (out of the hundred or so who tried out) were sitting in the office awaiting orders to BUD/S. Matt, me, and another guy. Why? Because we had removed temptation and prepared ourselves like crazy people on a radical mission, leaving little to chance.

> Resilience is not about hard work toward short-term gains, but rather maintaining the long-term grind toward an ultimate goal.

Nothing had stood in our way, especially not Temptation Tiger. But it was only the beginning.

Mental Model

Taming Temptation Tiger

The power to resist temptation has been extolled by philosophers, psychologists, teachers, coaches, and mothers. Anyone with advice on how you should live your life has surely spoken to you of its benefits. It is the path to a good life, professional and personal satisfaction, social adjustment, success, performance under pressure, and the best way for any child to avoid a Mom's icy stare over a very silent dinner. Of course, this assumes that our natural urges are a thing to be resisted—that there is a devil inside (or at the bottom of a cliff) luring you to cheat, offend, err, or indulge.

Why can't I keep myself from doing X? Why can't I accomplish Y? There are many possible reasons why we fail to resist temptation in our lives, but one of those answers is that we are not exercising *self-control*. You can't embrace the suck without it. Is this too simplistic? Given recent findings in psychology and some ancient philosophical thought, simple or not, for many people this is the key.

In the recent book *Willpower: Rediscovering the Greatest Human Strength*, Roy Baumeister and John Tierney discuss some of the psychological research related to the virtue of self-control. The book kicks off with the claim that research shows two qualities are consistently good predictors of success in achieving one's goals in life: *intelligence* and *self-control*. We may not be able to significantly increase our intelligence, and I would argue that point a bit, but we can increase our capacity for self-control. We can train it into ourselves.

The book discusses the muscle model of self-control. Each of us has a finite amount of willpower, which depletes as we use it. Also, we use the same stock of willpower for many tasks. If I use up most of my willpower during the day at work, I may have less self-control at night and be impatient with my wife and kids. This is the downside. Like a muscle, exertion results in fatigue. However, over the long term, a muscle that is consistently exercised increases in stamina and power. Fortunately, the same is true of self-control as it is for resilience. Like our comfort zone, our reserve of willpower can grow over time. Our capacity for self-control is benefitted by setting clear and realistic goals, by monitoring our progress toward those goals and sharing our successes and setbacks with others. When we exercise self-control, over time our willpower can increase in both stamina and impact. This is good news.

One way to cultivate self-control, for example, is to regularly exercise. In one longitudinal study, individuals who began an exercise program increased their self-control over a two-month period. They exhibited better self-control in behaviors that are both related and unrelated to exercise, as well as their performance on a self-control task in the laboratory. They watched less television; smoked fewer cigarettes; consumed less alcohol, caffeine, and junk food; engaged in less impulsive overspending; and procrastinated less often. In addition, they studied more, were more faithful in keeping their commitments, and reported an increase in their emotional control. The findings of this study suggest that our regulatory stock is not set; it can be increased by several behaviors.

> We become just by doing just actions, temperate by doing temperate actions, brave by doing brave actions.
>
> —ARISTOTLE

Practice doesn't make perfect, but it can make us better at resisting temptation and becoming the kind of people we want to and ought to be. Want to be more resilient? Practice the behaviors and decisions associated with resilience. Want to exercise better self-control? Start with small decisions and build from there.

Temptation isn't always about being lured down a dark path to do bad things. The modern world we live in is full of real-time messaging, distractions, and competing priorities. We are constantly inundated with alerts and communications from our many devices. Technology ensures we are always connected. And because of these advancements, our needs and expectations have changed. Constant distractions require us to be *more disciplined* than ever before.

Just like a responsible business leader has a specific mission plan with structured milestones and key performance indicators (KPIs), so too must those of us wishing to achieve specific personal goals. That mission plan is critical for maintaining focus on both the long-term vision and the path that gets us there. And there's nothing wrong with shifting the plan or changing our goals—in fact, sometimes it's absolutely necessary.

So, without further ado, I'd like to introduce you to the Taming Temptation Tiger mental model.

TAMING TEMPTATION TIGER

1 CLEARLY DEFINE YOUR GOALS
Write them down. Make them specific and time bound.

2 VISUALIZE WINNING
Visualize achieving your goal and work backward to define the road map.

3 LIST OBSTACLES
Identify behaviors, actions, tendencies, and people that stand in your way.

4 REMOVE ROADBLOCKS
This part sucks. Do it anyway. Eliminate the obstacles listed.

5 UNFUCK YOURSELF
Develop a plan for rapid course correction when you deviate.

Clearly Define Your Goals: We'll get more into goal setting and the planning process in later chapters, but it's necessary to touch on now as it relates to avoiding temptation and competing priorities. When we don't make our goals concise, time bound, measurable, and realistic (with a strategic plan to support each goal), it becomes much easier to allow distraction to derail progress. New shiny objects appear, and we start chasing "opportunities" unrelated to our goals and values.

Visualize Winning: Literally. Elite athletes and coaches do this. Special operators do it. Successful entrepreneurs do it. Great philanthropists. Oscar-winning actors. You name it. When we visualize the winning outcome and how we will arrive at that outcome, our brains begin working backward to define the path forward. If your goal is to run a marathon, then visualize yourself running the race and feeling the pain, the emotion, and the joy of the finish line. Picture each training day leading up to the race. What will you do? How will you feel? What temptations will you avoid?

List Obstacles: The best way to avoid temptations and distractions is to list them. Give them a name. Rank them based on your tendencies toward weakness in these areas. What threats and blockages stand in your way? What has caused you to fail in the past? If you tend to not finish projects you start, ask yourself the five whys of the Root Cause Analysis Model (page 53). Get to the root cause and label it.

Remove Roadblocks: Gradually begin managing these tendencies and removing obstacles. If you're stuck in a dead-end job or relationship, stop being so weak and get the fuck out. If you want to be a better leader for your team at work, make time to engage in personal and professional development. And yes, that means doing it at the expense of other enjoyable but time-wasting pursuits. Remove all rituals, activities, and behaviors that stand in your way—but don't do it at the expense of other people's well-being.

Unfuck Yourself: Have a plan for rapid course correction. Find an accountability partner, a trusted friend or colleague with whom you share your goals, objectives, challenges, and desired results. Schedule regular check-ins with your accountability partner and encourage them to keep you on track and be brutally honest when necessary. Get angry with yourself when weakness sets in. Or as David Goggins would say, "Go to war with yourself." Then unfuck yourself and course correct as needed.

Temptation is just a reality of life. Without it, there would be no such thing as willpower. Life will test you on a regular basis. So be prepared to ace the test!

Great, So What Now?

Finding magical opportunities beyond our comfort zone requires focus and follow-through. It also requires action-oriented thinking and resilience. As we continue to develop discipline and mental toughness, we will be more equipped to bounce back.

Mental fortitude and emotional intelligence are necessary for life beyond our comfort zone. They equip us with the battle gear for resisting temptation and crushing our goals.

Questions to ask yourself:

Do I stand tall in the face of temptation or allow the Tiger to pull me down the wrong path?

Upon reflection, what have I learned about previous failed attempts to resist temptation? How can I apply those lessons learned?

What are the top three temptations holding me back? Can I use the Taming Temptation Tiger mental model to attack those roadblocks with a vengeance?

If I know certain temptations hold me back from living a more fulfilling life, why haven't I changed those behaviors?

PART 2

GET COMFORTABLE BEING UNCOMFORTABLE

The only easy day was yesterday.
—NAVY SEAL PHILOSOPHY

5

IF YOU AIN'T FAILIN', YOU AIN'T TRYIN'

Every adversity, every failure, every heartache carries with it the seed of an equal or greater benefit.

—NAPOLEON HILL

Iraq
Enemy Target in a Rural Area Outside Baghdad
11:43 P.M.

So there I was, waist deep in shit. Literally. In life, things don't always go as planned, do they? Let me explain the events leading up to and following this shitty situation. Here are thirty-one steps to saying, *"Well that sure sucked!"*

Step 1: One of our Humvee's tires blows out on the way to the target. Stop. Throw in some chewing tobacco. Set security. Change tire.

Step 2: About a mile out from the target, the AC-130 Spectre gun-ship providing air support radios that people are moving on target.

Step 3: Arrive at target. Assault team inserts about one click (1,000 meters) from the target house and moves in on foot.

Step 4: We find not one but three structures on target. We reconfigure into a skirmish line and move through the target area, clearing one structure at a time.

Step 5: While moving toward a small structure with my squad, a four-man fire team, I maintain focus on the main door. As I move closer, I fall waist-deep into a cesspool. I'm covered in human shit. We were only a few minutes into the mission and it had already become a crappy situation.

Step 6: The AC-130 gunship radios that we have six squirters (people running off target) heading north. They drop several 40mm grenade rounds to stop the squirters' movement. One squad hops into a Humvee and races off to go round them up. The AC-130 talks them into the enemy location. It was just two women and four children—unharmed.

Step 7: We finish clearing the main target house, finding only one male. Not our guy.

Step 8: During our sensitive sight exploitation we encounter heavy resistance—from cows, goats, and llamas. They were not happy about our presence.

Step 9: We find dozens of SA-7s, AK-47s, RPGs, and grenades under large tarps in the small farmhouse. No bad guys, but at least we found the weapons cache.

Step 10: I'm still covered in human waste. It stinks.

Step 11: We load some of the weapons into the Humvees and pile the rest in the main house. Our explosive ordnance disposal (EOD) technician sets explosive charges to destroy the weapons.

Step 12: Before blowing the charges, we decide the humane thing to do is herd all of the enemy cows, goats, and llamas into a pen on the far side of the property so they don't get incinerated.

Step 13: Heavily armed Navy SEALs attempt to herd livestock. It does not go well. I specifically recall one of our guys—rifle slung—trying to drag a pissed off goat across the yard using a rope that had been placed around its neck. Hence the term "goat rope" (slang for "totally fucked up").

Step 14: Our lead breacher—a big-time cowboy—comes out of the house and takes over, successfully herding the animals into the pen like a pro. It was impressive.

Step 15: Pile into the vehicles and begin *exfil* off target. Charges blow, sending a giant fireball into the night sky.

Step 16: One of the vehicles—a $300,000 fully armored Mercedes G-Class carrying our agency guys and their source—goes off the road. The intel guy at the wheel had limited experience driving while wearing night vision goggles.

Step 17: The Mercedes is damaged and must be towed. While towing it behind one of the Humvees, the rural farm road narrows, and it rolls off into yet another ditch—with the agency guys and their source in the vehicle. It's now lying on its side in a six-foot-deep trench. Its occupants have to crawl out of the side windows.

Step 18: I'm still covered in human waste—but at least it's starting to dry.

Step 19: We secure cargo straps to the Mercedes, and are able to pull it right side up and out of the ditch using one of the Humvees.

Step 20: The convoy resumes exfil and starts heading back to base. The sun is now coming up. We enter an urban area and traffic is starting to pick up. Rush hour!

Step 21: The convoy increases speed (standard procedure in an urban area) and the Mercedes hits a curb and goes halfway off the side of a bridge. Unbelievable! It's now wedged into a smashed cement barrier.

Step 22: Convoy stops, we dismount, throw in some chewing tobacco, set security, and start directing traffic. Humvees attach cargo straps but can't budge the heavy SUV.

Step 23: I flag down a guy with a large cargo truck to help. He was reluctant, to say the least. Maybe it was my smelly pants that turned him off, not sure.

Step 24: For two more hours, we direct morning rush hour traffic and attempt to get the Mercedes off the side of the bridge. It's now 10 a.m. the following day. Already above 100 degrees.

Step 25: We eventually say screw it, remove radios and sensitive material, and leave the SUV behind. We would have to come back later and get it.

Step 26: We arrive back at base. I take off my disgusting pants and throw them in the pit where we burned our trash. I walk back to the tent in boxers and body armor. Fatigue sets in.

Step 27: A few of us and some Army brothers with a flatbed head back out to retrieve the Mercedes on loan from our agency partners.

Step 28: We arrive at the bridge only to find that some innovative individuals had been kind enough to dislodge the Mercedes from the side of the bridge. The only problem was that it was completely stripped! No doors. No wheels. Engine gone.

Step 29: Return to base.

Step 30: Write big check to agency partners.

Step 31: During the after-action review, you think, *well, that sure sucked.*

✪

My very first big stage speaking engagement was at the 2012 Inc. 500|5000 Conference and Awards in Phoenix, Arizona, in front of more than 600 people. This particular keynote was part of Inc.'s "vetrepreneur" celebration, which honors and supports military veteran business owners. Oh, and I was sharing the stage with none other than world-renowned speaker and author Simon Sinek. Which I found out upon arrival. No pressure at all. But, nervously I took the stage and did my thing. People clapped and that was that. No big deal. Easy day. My only priority was to connect with fellow veterans transitioning or starting businesses anyway. About a week later, I had a call with Eric Schurenberg, event emcee and editor-in-chief of *Inc.* magazine to debrief. Being the feedback-craving former SEAL that I am, I asked what he thought. Admittedly, I was teeing up "the ask" for speaking at future Inc. events—a potentially great way to generate brand awareness and thought leadership for my company at the time. After a brief pause of awkward silence, he said, "Well, Brent, it wasn't good. It just wasn't polished. You seemed unprepared. It was just kind of all over the place."

Bam! It was like a donkey kick to the face. Speaking was something I felt I could find a passion for, but clearly wasn't good at yet. And I hate losing far more than I enjoy winning. This felt like losing. I'm thinking, *B-b-b-b-but everyone clapped, and I think a couple people even stood up! Maybe they were going to the bathroom. I don't know. What does this guy know anyway?!* Surprise. Anger. Disappointment . . . then gradually, acceptance. Realization. Motivation. I vowed never to be unprepared again. I didn't realize it, but I had developed a growth mindset having endured both the rigors of SEAL training, combat, graduate school, and now the unforgiving battlefield of business and entrepreneurship. Now I speak, on average, fifty times a year all over the world and religiously maintain a very specific preparation process. Eric's feedback was painful at first, but it became a source of motivation. It was an awakening. As Winston Churchill once said, "Success is not final, failure is not fatal. It is the courage to continue that counts."

It was the same when the SEAL instructors would tell us that we should just quit. That training would only get worse—why put ourselves through all that? As a result, some would actually quit. They momentarily forgot that pain is temporary, but quitting is something that stays with you forever. Others found the fire in their gut necessary to carry on. Just enough fire to embrace the suck!

Before their rise to the top, some of the world's most successful people experience epic failure. We like to celebrate the success of the people we admire or envy but often overlook the path that got them there. It's a long road that is always marked with obstacles and failure. Their crowning achievements stem from drive and determination as much as from ability. Persistence and certitude provide the ammunition for combating failure.

As Thomas Edison once said, "I have not failed. I have only found ten thousand ways that something won't work." But let's face it. Failure sucks. Nobody sets out to fail or tells themselves, *Gee, I can't wait to take a fucking face-plant on this project, so I learn some valuable lessons.* Hell no. We don't tell ourselves we hope we get fired from our dream job so we can build some emotional and psychological resilience. We don't say, *Hey, I sure hope a global pandemic strikes so I can learn how to apply for government funding or unemployment.* The lessons learned come after the surprise, depression, disappointment, and anger wear off and enlightenment slowly starts to set in. *If* we choose to let it do so. If we apply lessons learned and vow to work our asses off to make incremental improvements over time.

There are endless examples. Oprah Winfrey is North America's first black multibillionaire, a world-renowned media mogul, and one of the greatest philanthropists in American history, but she was fired from her first TV job as an anchor in Baltimore for being—get this—too passionate about the stories. Jerry Seinfeld was booed off the stage many times early in his career, with close friends and family telling him to take life more seriously and choose a real career. As we all know, he is now one of the most famous comedians of all time. And can you imagine your childhood without Disney? Well, that could easily have been reality if Walt had listened to his former newspaper editor, who told Walt he "lacked imagination and had no good ideas." Undeterred, old Walt went on to create the cultural icon that bears his name. David Goggins grew up combating childhood obesity, depression, learning disorders, and abuse. Now he's a retired SEAL and known as one of the most elite extreme athletes in the world. All of these are perfect examples of a growth mindset.

They say that nothing breeds success like failure. Indeed, most of us eventually accept that failure is a reality of life, essential for growth even. But still we hate to fail. But why, when we intellectually acknowledge that failure can be turned into opportunity, are we so afraid of it? One of the models we teach leaders and business executives in our leadership and organizational development programs is Steven Kerr's simple performance formula. Kerr is a senior advisor to Goldman Sachs after a six-year term as a managing director and Goldman's chief learning officer (CLO). Before joining Goldman, he spent seven years as General Electric's CLO and vice president of corporate leadership development, working closely with Jack Welch and leading GE's renowned leadership education center. He went on to co-found the Jack Welch Management Institute. His formula is as follows:

$$Ability \times Motivation = Performance$$

Obviously, you can break ability and motivation down into many elements but overall, this is it. We use this model to help leaders better understand how to coach and mentor those on their team. If, for example, you have a direct report with high levels of ability and motivation in a given role, and then promote them into a new position, things might change in the near term. In a new role, they may be tackling challenges they have not faced, so their ability is lower. Sometimes people simply burn out regardless of ability and subject matter expertise, so motivation lessens as does performance. You get the idea.

Why is this a multiplication formula and not an addition formula? I'll pause for you to consider your answer....

Okay, time's up. Because if one factor is zero, performance equals zero. Also, known as *failure*. Most candidates arriving at BUD/S show up with both high levels of ability and motivation. That is, until they are put in situations they've never dealt with and placed in the most physically and mentally adverse scenarios of their lives. That's what makes the training program a very level playing field. Sure, some students are rock star runners or swim like dolphins. High ability and motivation results in high performance in those specific evolutions. But when tested in other areas, that's often not the case. Meanwhile, others seem to be totally averse to pain and stress, but struggle in various pass-fail evolutions that require focus and technical ability.

Each phase in BUD/S has pass-fail evolutions. In most, the student is only given one or two chances. If failure is the result, they're packing their bags—*"haze gray and underway"*—off to the fleet. The first evolution is the fifty-meter underwater swim.

The students line up along the side of the Olympic-size swimming pool at the Naval Amphibious Base across the street from the Naval Special Warfare Center. They jump in feet first, do an underwater somersault (which can cause you to blow too much precious air from your lungs), and without pushing off the wall, swim down and back for a total of fifty meters. Sometimes heads break the surface early gasping for air or students pass out before reaching the wall. Fail! Devastation soon follows.

Another wonderful evolution is called drownproofing. The student's arms are tied behind his back and his ankles are tethered together. He must then perform a series of exercises like swimming multiple laps for hundreds of meters, bobbing up and down in the deep end, and swimming down five meters to pick up a swim mask off the bottom of the pool with his teeth. This goes on for a long time. If you aren't very comfortable in the water or motivated enough to find the resilience to dig deep, failure is imminent.

Some students who have dreamed of these moments their whole lives have those dreams shattered in a matter of minutes. And there are no participation trophies handed out. Some can try again months or years later and succeed. Some are never seen or heard from again.

But Everyone Gets a Trophy, Right?

The two youngest of our three children (a six-year-old daughter and a four-year-old son) played soccer last year. Let's just say their level of commitment and performance could have been better. I get it, they are very young, and I sound like an asshole, but I'm trying to make a point. Our son Ryder's main coach held a small trophy ceremony after the last game of the season. He handed out the trophies one at a time, telling a brief story about each player. Ryder's turn came around.

"Okay, who's up next? Can any of you guys tell me who this next trophy goes to? I'll give you a hint . . . he likes to aimlessly walk the field while eating chicken fingers during the game," his coach said in that tone you use when talking to four-year-olds. You had to be there, but during one of his games, when he was on the field of battle, he was wandering around eating a giant chicken finger. It was pretty hysterical. But the SEAL in me yearned for just a bit higher level of accountability and performance.

Three of the kids on Ryder's team immediately shot their hands up saying, "Ryder, it was Ryder!" Ryder proudly rose and accepted his well-earned trophy. It was his first badge of honor signifying weeks of dedication, hard work, and discipline on and off the battlefield! He was so excited and utterly pleased with himself; the whole car ride home he kept joyfully exclaiming in a squeaky voice, "My first trophy ever! Can you believe it?!" As soon as we got home, I took the trophy away and told him, "We don't reward mediocrity in this house." He immediately burst into tears.

I'm kidding, of course. I congratulated him yet again and then helped him find a prominent place for it on the shelf in his room. Then cooked up some chicken fingers.

At what point do we start teaching our children to embrace the suck? And how about failure? When is it too early? When is it too late?

The Science of Failure

According to Professor Martin Covington of the University of California, Berkeley, the fear of failure is directly linked to our sense of self-worth. His research on students, published in the *Handbook of Motivation at School,* found that one of the ways we protect our self-worth is by believing we are competent and by convincing others of it too. For this reason, the ability to achieve is critical in maintaining self-worth. To fail to perform essentially means that we are not able and, therefore, not worthy.

Professor Covington found that if a person doesn't believe they have the ability to succeed (or if repeated failures diminish that belief), then they will engage in other practices that seek to preserve their self-worth. Often, these practices take the form of excuses or defense mechanisms. They regress back to—or stay— in a fixed mindset that reduces motivation and therefore ability to perform.

When it comes to dealing with failure, the professor grouped students into one of four categories:

Success-Oriented Students: These people are typically life-long learners and see failure as a way to improve as opposed to proof of their crappy self-worth.

Over-Strivers: Professor Covington calls these students "closet-achievers." They are so fearful of failing that they avoid it at all costs, even if it means exerting themselves beyond what is reasonably expected.

Failure-Avoiding Students: These students don't even expect to succeed. But they also simultaneously dread failing, so they do the bare minimum or try to blend in. In BUD/S, the instructors called this being the "gray man." This strategy never works.

Failure-Accepting Students: These people have basically already accepted defeat and failure as their reality. These students are very difficult to motivate. Seeing failure as inextricably connected to our sense of self-worth—or lack thereof—puts it in perspective. "By making our self-worth contingent on categories such as academic success, appearance, or popularity, we fail to value ourselves solely for the fact that we are human beings and accept that failure is part of the human experience," the professor explains.

Mental Model
How to Win at Failing

Failure is usually a fairly demoralizing and upsetting experience. It can alter your perception and make you believe things that simply aren't true. Unless you learn to respond to failure in psychologically adaptive ways, it can paralyze you, demotivate you, and limit your likelihood of success moving forward.

The Embrace the Suck model has Eight Failure Realities that you must understand in order to get comfortable being uncomfortable.

Reality 1: Failure makes the same goal seem less attainable. In one study at a special operations sniper school, instructors had the students fire at targets from the same distance on an unmarked range. They then had the students estimate the distance to the targets. Students who scored lower (fewer target hits than others) believed the targets to be significantly farther out than students who scored the highest. Failure distorts perception if you allow it to. The good news is that there are ways to avoid this.

Reality 2: Failure alters your perception of your abilities. As much as failure can distort your perception of goals, it can also alter your assumptions about ability. I've seen students who quit BUD/S or fail the selection process fall into deep depression—sometimes even become suicidal—while others come back a second or third time over the course of years and ultimately succeed. Failure can make us doubt our skills, intelligence, desirability, and capabilities. Simply acknowledging this is the first step to self-correction.

Reality 3: Failure can make you feel helpless. According to psychologists, this is a mental defense mechanism. When we fail, the brain sends signals making us feel temporarily helpless; it's an emotional wound so to speak. Like when a toddler touches a hot stove—the brain says, "Whoa buddy, don't do that shit again." The same applies with failure. When we allow ourselves to be convinced that we are helpless, we successfully avoid future failures. But that's actually what makes you a failure—when you listen to the voices and rob yourself of future success.

Reality 4: A failure experience can cause a fear of failure complex. People can also trend toward avoiding success as much as they try to avoid failure, but the two usually go hand-in-hand. Success rarely comes without some failure along the way, which makes the journey very uncomfortable. So rather than working on improving their ability, skills, or approach to succeeding at something, people head back to home base—their own cozy little comfort zone.

Reality 5: Fear of failure often leads to unconscious self-sabotaging. Like the college student who decides to stay out drinking until 2:00 a.m. before a big job interview he "knows" he'll bomb. Or the young kid who doesn't pick up a sport as naturally as her peers, so she tells her parents she hates it and wants to quit. These kinds of behaviors can turn into self-fulfilling prophecies and increase potential for future failure. But the best accomplishments in life usually reside on the other side of fear.

Reality 6: The pressure to succeed increases performance anxiety, causing choking. Choking at those critical gaming-winning moments. Blanking out during the test after weeks of studying. Leaving out the most critical talking points in your big speech. Usually, all of this is a result of simply over-thinking. This is why *proper* preparation is the bedrock of achievement and the most powerful tool for overcoming performance anxiety.

Reality 7: Willpower is like a muscle—it needs both training and rest. As we've discussed, much like muscles that become fatigued, mental willpower can become overworked and undernourished. Soldiers participating in sustained combat experience battle fatigue, which causes clouded thinking, lack of ability to control emotion, confusion, depression, and inhibited decision-making ability. So when you feel your willpower fading, be sure to rest and be willing to revisit your motivations once you've nourished your willpower muscles. Just don't rest too long!

Reality 8: The healthiest psychological response to failure is focusing on what you can control. This ability is a fundamental tenet of building resilience. Failure can result in us focusing primarily on the cause of our current adversity. We look backward instead of forward. We focus on the elements we have no control over as opposed to developing an action plan— leveraging what is in our control.

✪

Mark Owen, one of my closest friends, former teammate, team leader of a tier one NSW special missions unit, and author of the number one *New York Times* best-seller *No Easy Day*, told me a training story about reality number eight. Years ago, some guys from his squadron were participating in a lead climbing course outside of Las Vegas. In this rock climbing style, the lead climber must ascend various sections of the route in order to place "protection" in the case of a fall. That, of course, means that if you climb fifteen feet above your last piece of protection and fall, you'll be plummeting thirty feet before the rope catches you with a violent jolt, which sucks.

Mark was about eighty feet up and roughly twenty feet above his last piece of protection when he froze. He didn't trust his footholds and couldn't find his next move. Within seconds, his teammates noticed from below and the taunting and jeering began. The climbing instructor, a wiry little guy in board shorts and climbing shoes figured he'd use this as a coaching moment, so he lit a cigarette and started scaling the rock face—without a rope. In no time at all he reached Mark, still frozen against the wall. "What's up, bro?" the instructor inquired.

Mark looked down at his teammates who were still making fun of him. Then he looked out to the Vegas skyline. "Why are you looking down at the guys? They can't fucking help you. Neither can Las Vegas. Stay in your three-foot world bro. Right here. Only focus on what's in your immediate control. Ignore everything else," he said.

Maintaining focus on what is in our control and ignoring (or at least deprioritizing) everything else is a core tenet of the growth mindset and applies equally in achieving goals and overcoming obstacles in our personal and professional lives.

When I hung up my sword and stepped off the battlefield, I immediately began graduate school. This was part of my military transition strategy to retrain my brain toward business. At the time, entrepreneurship wasn't even a path I had considered. Later, during the program, our finance professor assigned group projects. You know, the kind of projects where two people do all the work and the other three drink beer. Yes, that kind. Well, while some of us were kicking back drinking beer we had an epiphany! It was a white space that had great potential, like with all entrepreneurs' brilliant ideas, right? Long story short, that project became the foundation of the business plan for my first company, a home finding search engine. We were to become entrepreneurs who'd retire at 35. Masters of our own destiny! The less brave comfort zone wanderers would envy us, watching our rise to the top while they grinded away at their mediocre jobs working for the man. Tales of glory and unprecedented success would echo for eternity. It would be outstanding!

Upon graduation, we hit the fundraising trail, expecting to bat away angel investors and venture capital firms right and left. I mean, I was a Navy SEAL for crying out loud. Who *wouldn't* throw money at this? At this point, I hope you're picking up on my sarcasm. We quickly realized that this whole entrepreneurship thing is fucking hard and super risky. There was a lot more suck-embracing than anticipated. Simply put, the failure rate for start-ups is the same if not higher than the failure rate for SEAL training candidates. But what the hell, if you ain't failin', you ain't tryin'!

Ultimately, we raised millions and that business—and others to follow—were successful. But not without a road riddled with the pockmarks of micro-failures, costly mistakes, and salty tears. My tears. The recession didn't help either. Didn't see that shit coming—despite my econ professor's many warnings. But this was a different battlefield and I was ill-trained in sniffing out the inevitable ambush. Obstacle after obstacle, I learned to focus on what was in my control and worry less about what wasn't. I learned to stay in my three-foot world.

Mitigating Failure Through Calculated Risk

So how the hell do we know when we are taking *calculated risk* versus *blind dumb risk*? Simple. When the crazy shit we decide to do turns into a positive outcome! I quit my lucrative job to join the Navy to try out for a program that has the highest attrition rate in the US military. Then, of course, came 9/11 and risks that followed. Know how many combat missions I've been on with very limited intel? More than a couple! Then I dove headfirst into entrepreneurship with no money, no income, and a condo I couldn't afford. Several years later, I met my unbelievably amazing wife at a wedding in Costa Rica. We got matching tattoos four weeks after meeting. Obviously. Oh, and then we got married a couple months later. And, yes, we are still married!

So in retrospect we can go back and label risky decisions as calculated by saying, "We just knew we were meant to be together" or "Failure wasn't an option" and stuff like that. But wouldn't it be nice to have a model to follow so we can better weigh the potential outcomes and necessary contingencies when the unforeseen occurs? Of course it would.

We can pull from part of the goal setting and strategic planning frameworks we will dive into later, which are designed to tackle risk and mitigate failure.

Define the Goal. Such as marrying the girl you just met, taking down a terrorist stronghold with limited information, finally telling your unappreciative boss to fuck off, or launching yourself from a perfectly good airplane. Make the goal as concise, measurable, achievable, and time bound as possible.

List Threats and Hazards. *Don't really know the girl, could end badly. Unknown number of terrorists on target. Will probably get fired when I tell my boss to fuck off. Parachute may not open.* You'll come back to this list when weighing your options.

Identify Resources for Successful Execution. *Need to buy a ring. Shit, need money. Should probably ask her dad's approval. Need Spectre gunship for air support. Need backup job ASAP. Need properly packed parachute—and some skydiving lessons.*

Assess Go/No-Go Criteria. Use the information at hand to make the best possible decision to proceed—or not. Do the risks outweigh the resources and rewards? Be careful about getting advice from others. Ensure your sources are trusted and as unbiased as possible. But in my experience, when you're about to toss yourself willingly into the unknown oblivion of risk, everyone tells you not to proceed. Sometimes you gotta say fuck it and go with your gut. And remember The Three Ps!

Always Debrief. Somewhere down the road, assuming your decision was to move forward, it's important to debrief the execution and outcome. What went well? What didn't? What unforeseen events cropped up that I didn't have contingencies for? How did I respond? How will I execute better next time? Document your findings and refer back to them the next time you're about to charge the hill.

Great, So What Now?

Seeking the magical opportunities beyond your comfort zone will be paved with small (and sometimes large) setbacks. But failure can be one of life's greatest gifts. And who doesn't like a good gift every now and then? Calculate the risks and potential rewards.

Ask yourself how much regret you're willing to carry for *not* pushing the boundaries of your comfort zone.

Questions to ask yourself:

How do I respond in the face of failure and setbacks?

What could I potentially gain by looking at failure through a different lens?

Does failure drive my goals further away, or like Thomas Edison, just confirm a few ways things won't work?

How often do I assess the odds and take calculated risk?

How might I feel toward the end of my life if I realize I never really strayed from my comfort zone?

6

DO SOMETHING
THAT SUCKS EVERY DAY

Do something that sucks every day.
—DAVID GOGGINS

Sounds strange. "Do something that sucks every day." David Goggins's philosophy on mastering your mind is simple: push the boundaries of your comfort zone daily, mentally and physically. Psychological and physical fortitude require training—they are perishable qualities. Our comfort zones are surrounded by moveable barriers. When we take decisive action in pushing against those barriers, our comfort zones begin to overflow with challenges, tasks, and fears we used to deem insurmountable. They become part of our everyday lives. Whether it be obstacles at work, difficult relationships unattended to, goals unaccomplished, or fears not faced, the more you lean in, the more you score. Then you move the goalposts and do it again.

As he mentioned in the foreword, David Goggins and I met in the fall of 2000 at BUD/S. We had both been assigned to class 235. He was an intimidating beast of a guy who didn't smile much. Okay, never. He'd already been through Hell Week twice due to injuries. No wonder he wasn't smiling. I have heard David say numerous times, "Life fucking sucks. Get over it." His experiences are captured in his best-selling book *Can't Hurt Me*.

Later in life, driven by the notion of giving to a cause greater than himself, David applied to join the United States Air Force Pararescue. He failed his ASVAB (Armed Services Vocational Aptitude Battery) twice before he succeeded and entered Pararescue training. He then became a member of the United States Air Force Tactical Air Control Party, also known as TACP—we love our acronyms. He served his time in TACP and left the United States Air Force to return to civilian life. He ended up with a job as an exterminator, regained excess weight, and fell into a deep depression. The demons of his past returned to haunt him, pulling him further into the depths.

One day, David looked in the mirror and told himself that he refused to live that life. That he would not be a slave to his sordid past. He still had a passion for military service, so he decided to step up his game and go to the local Navy recruiter's office. He told them he planned to try out for the SEAL program. At the time, David was 6'1" and 297 pounds. The recruiters discouraged him from even attempting, saying he needed to lose at least forty pounds. So, David went home. Two months later he returned, having lost a significant amount of weight and in amazing condition. He still needed to trim down more, but he figured BUD/S would take care of that.

David succeeded in graduating from training (after doing Hell Week three times) with my class in 2001, and we were both assigned to SEAL Team Five. But this was not enough. Not enough sacrifice, not enough purposeful suffering. During his second platoon cycle, he attended the elite Army Ranger School and graduated as the Top Honor Man. Ranger school comes with its own unique set of challenges, and David was not ordered to do so—he had requested to go.

After many of our brothers made the ultimate sacrifice in Afghanistan in 2005 during Operation Red Wings, he began long-distance running to raise money for the Special Operations Warrior Foundation. The Foundation gives college scholarships and grants to the children of fallen special operations soldiers. What do I mean by long-distance? I mean one hundred miles or more.

David sat down one day and typed "hardest ultramarathons in the world" into the Google search bar. Yep, that's how his mind works. Why start small? He found the Badwater 135, notably one of the most challenging races known to man. He attempted to enter as a fundraiser, but organizers told him that he needed to enter another ultramarathon first and finish with a qualifying time, as the Badwater is an invitation-only event. Literally two days later, with no training, he signed up for the San Diego One Day, a 24-hour ultramarathon held at Hospitality Point in San Diego. David had never even run a 26.2-mile marathon, but he was able to run 101 miles in nineteen hours and six minutes.

Soon after, David completed his first marathon (Las Vegas), in a time that qualified him for entrance into the Boston Marathon. After those two events, having yet to be invited to the Badwater 135, he entered the HURT100, an ultramarathon in Hawaii that is widely regarded as one of the hardest ultramarathons in the world. He was ninth to cross the finish line—only twenty-three runners completed the course. He was pissed he didn't win. He was subsequently granted entry into the 2006 Badwater 135. He finished fifth overall, an unheard-of result for an ultramarathon novice. Sure, we run a lot in the SEAL Teams, but not 100 miles. That's what helicopters and Humvees are for!

You see, David is driven by a fire that burns deep inside his soul. It's a fire, in large part, fueled by adversity. We all have that flame. Not everyone's is derived from extreme hardship or abuse, but we either choose to use it to our advantage or we ignore it. David continues to do something that sucks every day. As I write this, he is completing the five-day Moab 240. "I need to recertify myself as a savage," he said in an interview. If that's not the epitome of a growth mindset, I don't know what is.

We don't all have to run 240 miles to be a savage every day. It's up to us how we choose to define what being a badass means.

★

Another world-class runner who experienced more adversity and suffering than you or I could possibly fathom? Meet good old Louis Zamperini. His greatest obstacle was his own mortality—you'll know what I mean in a minute. His story of resilience is captured in Laura Hillenbrand's number one *New York Times* best-seller *Unbroken: A World War II Story of Survival, Resilience, and Redemption*. During World War II, his entire focus was on surviving, and the odds continued to stack against him. He joined the Air Force in 1941 and was stationed in the Pacific as a bombardier on a B-24 Liberator bomber. At that time, flying into combat was only half the danger. Due to numerous technical problems and inadequate training, more than 50,000 airmen died in noncombat-related accidents. So it was not an unusual occurrence when Louis's plane crashed into the ocean as he and his crewmates flew on a search-and-rescue mission for another plane that went down earlier that day.

What was unusual, however, was that Louis survived the crash and the subsequent forty-seven days he spent on a raft. Starvation. Sharks. Strafing by enemy fighter planes. Extreme thirst. Hallucinations. Death. "The odds of being rescued if you ended up on a life raft were terrible," Laura Hillenbrand told NPR in 2010. "The rafts were very poorly equipped." Louis and his crewmate survived at sea longer than any other known survivors, drinking rainwater and eating the fish they managed to catch. They were regularly attacked by Japanese fighter planes forcing them to dive into shark-infested waters.

But his struggle to survive had only just begun. Believe it or not, things were about to get worse. There would be a lot more suck to embrace. Emaciated and weak from floating around the Pacific for a month and a half, Louis was captured by the Japanese and eventually sent to a brutal POW camp where he was beaten, starved, and overworked.

Unfortunately for Louis, he also happened to be a world-famous Olympian. Who would have thought that this could get him into trouble? But it did. He had competed in the 1936 Olympics and was one of the fastest distance runners in the world. A jealous and sadistic prison guard, Mutsuhiro Watanabe—whom the prisoners nicknamed "The Bird"—singled out Louis for particularly cruel treatment. This guy was a real entitled asshole, and he developed a bizarre obsession with Louis.

These events are dramatized in the movie *Unbroken*, based on Laura's best-selling book. Amazingly, Louis survived two years in the POW camp before being released at the end of the war. He was the ultimate savage, never broken. Finally at home, he was free and no longer living under the threat of torture and death every day. But now he faced a new and unexpected obstacle: living with the trauma of the past two years and the inescapable memories of the brutal treatment he received. "Louis came home a deeply, deeply haunted man," Laura says. Once his physical needs were finally met and the brutality of the war was over, Louis had to confront his invisible scars.

Every night he would wake up screaming from horrible nightmares about the cruel guard who had tried to break his spirit and nearly killed him. His thoughts would return to his horrific experiences and he would relive the beatings in his mind. Coping with the traumas of the past—what would now be diagnosed as Post-Traumatic Stress Disorder (PTSD)—was an obstacle he had not prepared for. He began abusing alcohol and soon his marriage began to suffer (he married Cynthia Applewhite shortly after returning home).

Fortunately, true to his resilient spirit, Louis found ways to overcome this new obstacle, just as he overcame the odds during the war. He overcame PTSD and went on to live nearly seventy more fruitful and happy years, free from the terrors of the past.

Of course, this wasn't suffering he chose. He did, however, choose how to react. So where did this resilience come from? His family moved to Torrance, California, in 1919, where Louis attended Torrance High School. He and his family spoke no English when they moved to California, making him a target for bullies because of his Italian roots. He regularly found himself in fights. His father had taught him how to box, so he soon found an interest in brawling. His older brother, a high school track star, convinced him to join the cross-country team in an attempt to save him from his downward spiral. He quickly found a passion for running and channeled his inner rage (the flame) into positive aggression.

He developed resilience that ultimately saved his life.

Mental Model
Practicing the Things That Suck

Stress and anxiety can be great tools if you know how to use them. If you choose to use them. With all the media and medical attention on the negative impacts of stress, it's easy to conclude that it's irredeemably bad, something to be avoided at all costs. This applies to both physical and emotional stress and anxiety.

I have a different perspective, as do many psychologists who are well versed in this field. Pursuing a stress-free life often causes more stress down the road; problems compound and when we fail to face our greatest challenges, we never overcome them. The same applies for comfort zone expansion—the challenges and suffering we choose to pursue. If David hadn't joined the Air Force, he probably would have never become a SEAL. If he hadn't become a SEAL, he definitely wouldn't have started running insanely miserable 240-mile races (it's not for everyone). He wouldn't get to experience the joy of suffering for something meaningful—supporting our warriors and motivating people all over the world. He'd be safe, depressed, and overweight in his mediocre comfort zone.

Think about a time when you experienced substantial personal and professional growth, or a time when you performed at your highest level. Say finishing a race. Building a business—or saving a struggling business. Being accepted to your reach school.

Landing your dream job. Or raising a child. What was it that motivated and fueled you to grow, learn, and improve during these experiences? I'm willing to bet those times invariably involved some stress, suffering, and struggle.

Drawing on their work and research with executives, Navy SEALS, students, and professional athletes, behavioral psychologists Alia Crum and Thomas Crum developed a three-step model for responding to pressure and harnessing the creative power of stress while minimizing its deleterious effects.

The model is simple and looks like this:

STEP ONE: See it.

We typically only stress about things we give a shit about. It shows we care. When we can start labeling that stress, the solutions for navigating it become far more apparent. For example, on the days I'm feeling stressed out or experiencing some anxiety, I ask my wife, *Why the hell am I so stressed*? The intention is not necessarily for her to answer the question. Though when she does, she's always right. It's a method for me to break down the possible root causes and identify them. And usually it's not what I initially think and totally unrelated to what's actually consuming my thoughts.

Neuroscience research from Matthew Lieberman of UCLA shows how just acknowledging stress and adversity can move reactivity in your brain from the automatic and reactive centers to the more conscious and deliberate ones. For example, therapists who work with veterans suffering from PTSD use a desensitization method that gets to the root cause of the trauma, which is usually a very specific event. This allows the person to acknowledge it, see it, and eventually move past it.

STEP TWO: Own it.

As I mentioned, we usually only stress about things that matter to us. Owning this realization unleashes that positive aggression I keep referring to, because deep down we know that the things that really matter in life don't come easy.

As a board member of the SEAL Family Foundation I often give potential donors tours of the BUD/S training facility. One attendee asked a great question of the SEAL instructor assisting with the tour. "So what's the secret sauce? How do you take regular guys and turn them into elite warriors that can overcome almost any amount of adversity?" The answer was even better than the question.

"In SEAL training, the instructor cadre design situations that can be exponentially more stressful, chaotic, and dynamic than a combat operation so that the team learns to center themselves in the most arduous circumstances. When the stress of the training seems unbearable, we can own it, knowing that ultimately it is what we have chosen to do—to be a member of a team and win in any situation."

Basically, we do something that sucks every day, so we get comfortable being uncomfortable.

STEP THREE: Use it.

Though it often feels like it, the body's stress response was not designed to kill us. In fact, the evolutionary goal of the stress response was to help boost the body and mind into enhanced functioning, to help us grow and meet the demands we face. Louis knew that if he wanted to become the fastest man in the world, pain, stress, and suffering would be a regular gateway to victory. If he wanted to survive torture and starvation, he'd have to dig deep.

And while the stress response can sometimes have adverse effects, in many cases, stress hormones do in fact induce growth and release chemicals into the body that rebuild cells, synthesize proteins, and enhance immunity, leaving the body even stronger and healthier. Researchers call this effect physiological thriving, and any athlete, combat veteran, or POW survivor knows its rewards. As we have discussed, it's all about perspective. Shifting the narrative on anxiety to excitement and opportunity can improve performance on any task or objective.

How to Do Something That Sucks Every Day

It's difficult for most of us to compare ourselves to people like David and Louis, world-class athletes, top scholars and musicians, astronauts and award-winning rodeo clowns. Living an extraordinary life means something different to all of us based on our values and goals. We must first define what a winning outcome looks like, then work backward to design the intricate web of pathways that will connect us to fulfilling that prophecy.

The challenge is that we often engage in activities that have no real connection to our passions, purpose, values, or goals. It's about doing the *right* things that suck. People choose jobs that leave them unfulfilled. Stay in relationships that will only end in suffering. Hold grudges that only cause more pointless pain. Follow paths defined by others, which are rarely the paths less traveled. Get caught up in hateful acts for no real reason. Become distracted by laziness and temptation and give up on fitness goals. Quit when the going gets tough.

So how do you do the right things that suck every day in order to overcome adversity, exceed your goals, and live an extraordinary life? Let's start here. We will apply this later when covering your personal mission plan and execution strategy.

List Your Top Twenty Personal and Professional Goals: These should be two different lists, but keep in mind how these two areas of focus will impact the other. There is really no such thing as work-life balance. Its work-life *integration*. Listing twenty goals sounds like a daunting task, but let's do it anyway.

Narrow the List Down to Five or Six Goals: So, after all that, I'm asking you to cut fourteen or fifteen goals? Yes, I am. Really consider the goals that have true meaning to you. Reflect on your passions. Your true purpose in life. Your values. Which goal would have you leaping out of bed every morning ready to kick ass and take names? Which goals might have a positive impact on others? Anything else is a distraction.

Define the Actions Necessary to Achieve Each Goal: Make a list of five or six specific actions (let's not worry about the time-bound nature of these activities yet). Reflect on each action and identify elements that make you uncomfortable. Again, as I previously mentioned, the most meaningful goals that will provide the greatest satisfaction will have aspects that make you cringe.

Start Practicing the Things That Suck: Okay, now you have five or six personal and professional goals, each with one or two things that suck assigned to them. Make a list. Put it on your desk, anywhere it's visible on a regular basis. Take every opportunity to practice, practice, practice. If you want to compete in an Ironman but aren't comfortable in the water, you better start swimming. You get the idea.

What do I mean by practice? SEALs are arguably the best at what we do in our given field. Yet we practice, rehearse, dirt dive, execute, and debrief constantly. Over and over. The general public might assume SEALs are constantly deployed downrange, but we actually spend 75 percent of our time training. The other 25 percent of the time we are deployed. And on deployment, when we aren't fighting, eating, or sleeping, we're training—living each day in a constant state of improvement.

When I began seriously training for the BUD/S program well before joining the Navy, I'd lost much of my endurance for long-distance swimming and running. Sure I had been a college athlete, but just a year working in corporate America had robbed me of my stamina. I struggled with the longer runs, often falling way behind my buddy with whom I was training. That really pissed me off. During the first few sessions at the SMU pool, just swimming 100 meters seemed like crossing the English Channel. I hadn't swum competitively in years. I was nowhere near being prepared for the BUD/S entrance PT test. Outside of research and designing a very specific training regime (all of which sucked big time) my vow was simple: puke during or after every workout, push the limits every time.

I know it sounds a bit stupid and barbaric, but it worked. I knew I would never be prepared and make the gains in short- and long-term strength and endurance necessary unless I made myself suffer. I planned to mark fitness off my list of concerns, and that was the only way. That piece was in my control. One day,

I was training at the SMU track. Suddenly, Olympic champion sprinter Michael Johnson walks onto the field. Just me and MJ. I wasn't going to let the fact that he was the fastest man in the world discourage me! Let's just say I puked a lot that afternoon.

If one of your personal goals is related to fitness, I recommend creating your own Wheel of Misfortune packed with exercises and routines designed to train you in key areas—you know, the ones you hate the most. One of my professional goals is to transform people and organizations through enhanced leadership ability at every level. That means I must constantly study and practice the art and science of leadership. One of the things on my list of stuff that sucks is having difficult conversations. On the literal battle-field, I ran swiftly to the sound of gunfire. In my current personal and professional life, however, I struggle with conflict avoidance. Tackling challenges and difficult conversations is critical for effective leadership. So, I make a point to practice, practice, practice. And it gets a little easier every time.

Military leaders make tough decisions every day. It takes some serious getting used to. Especially when those decisions put their own team members in harm's way. Unfortunately, these leaders have plenty of opportunity to practice. The point is, ultimately, once you have clearly defined goals, you know what stands in your way. The question is, how bad do you want to conquer those goals?

How willing are you to embrace the suck?

Great, So What Now?

Now it's time to start practicing the fine art of getting comfortable being uncomfortable. Comfort zone expansion is impossible without the consistent execution of this process. Over time, you'll find that not only does the discomfort dissipate, but you begin to enjoy many of the activities and obstacles you used to loathe. Then you make a new list and violently execute.

We cloak ourselves in mediocrity when we are unwilling embrace the challenges that stand in our way of greatness. So, use the models in this chapter to expedite your voyage to deeper levels of mental fortitude.

Questions to ask yourself:

What do I do regularly to at least peek over the barriers of my comfort zone? When I do, what do I see? Does it compel me to leap over or climb back down?

How do I channel the negative energy from adverse situations? Do I reinvest that energy into something new?

What positive benefits could come if I started doing something that sucks every day? What is my growth potential?

Am I committed to tackling the list of things that suck, knowing it will drive me closer to my goal?

7

CHOOSE WISELY WHAT YOU SUFFER FOR

> *Out of suffering have emerged the strongest*
> *souls; the most massive characters are seared*
> *with scars.*
>
> —KAHLIL GIBRAN

Iraq
1:13 A.M.

Panting vigorously, we ascended the stairs of the high-rise apartment. Apparently, it's not "tactical" or "sneaky" to cram a bunch of heavily armed operators into an elevator. So up we went, heading to the fourteenth floor. Our mission: kidnap or kill two high value enemy targets. Our task unit had broken into three teams—two assault units and one mobility unit providing exterior security. The mission plan called for two simultaneous breaches. One apartment was on the second floor while the other was on the fourteenth. We had drawn the short straw on this one, and boy were we suffering as we moved swiftly up the stairwell. Me especially.

I was sweating profusely—not so much from the exertion and weight of my kit, but from the wonderful 103-degree fever baking my brain. I had a horrible flu, or food poisoning, or both. Not sure. But it sucked. *I shouldn't have eaten that fucking lamb, or whatever it was at the meeting with that sheik yesterday,* I thought. My stomach was in knots. I'd spent most of the day in a fly-infested oven of a porta potty. I'll spare you the details.

The two apartments were housed in one of three seventeen-story buildings that were part of the complex set in a U-shaped configuration. All apartments were accessed by exterior hallways, kind of like a huge motel. We hit the fourteenth floor and moved stealthily down the breezeway. The tantalizing stench of diesel fuel, burning trash, and human waste permeated the air. We found the apartment and stacked along the exterior wall as the breacher set the explosive charge. I loved this dude. Remember the guy who herded the goats and llamas into the pin for us on that goat rope of an op? He was a good old boy from Texas who spent his day either working out or making breaching charges, safely tucked behind the walls of his private bomb-making room.

He crept back to our position ten feet from the door. We radioed the other team, passing the word that we were set and ready. This would be a simultaneous breach. They confirmed. "Charge is set. Three. Two. One. Execute," our breacher whispered.

BOOM!!! The concussion of the two blasts was so extreme it shattered nearly all the windows in all three high-rise towers. It was surreal. But that's not all it destroyed. As glass from the apartment windows just above our heads vaporized—sending the crystalized dust spraying in all directions—I felt a concussive blast of my own. *Oh shit!*

If you've ever assaulted an enemy target with diarrhea streaming down your legs, you may recall that it's not super cool. And you certainly don't feel like a badass Navy SEAL operator—more like an embarrassed preschooler on the playground. Nevertheless, we surged forward, peeling right and left into the apartment. The blast had destroyed the front living room. Luckily no noncombatants were injured. We flowed into the hallway to the left of the main room. An enemy fighter pulled a "spray and pray" maneuver— sticking his AK-47 around the corner from the room he was hiding in, sending massive bullets aimlessly down the corridor in our direction. The 7.62 rounds pounded the walls, each thankfully missing their intended target. We moved rapidly toward the burst of fire, tossed a grenade in the room, then finished our clearance, finding the high value target hiding in a back room. Our HVT now in custody, we radioed the other team. The other assault unit soon let us know they had their guy in custody. Two minutes later, we were climbing back into our vehicles. I was a prisoner handler, so I had our HVT secured in the back of one of the Humvees.

"Bro, did you crap your pants?" one of my teammates asked with a look of disgust on his face while flipping his night vision goggles up onto his helmet. "Yeah, asshole. I did." Naturally, a roar of laughter ensued. "Fuck off, I'm sick," I said annoyed and exhausted. My pants and top were soaked in sweat. We were ready to exfil off target. I couldn't wait to get back to our compound and toss my pants in the burn pit. Again! But no such luck.

"Gents, we just got spun up for another op," our platoon commander called out. *You've got to be kidding me!* After a quick mission brief, we piled back into our Humvees and Chevy Suburbans and headed out to the next target, a house about thirty minutes way. The guys smirked as they scooted away from me in the back of the Hummer. "Bro, you stink!" they laughed. The other target was a dry hole. No bad guys. Four hours later, we finally arrived back at our base. I shot out of the Humvee and headed straight for the burn pit. I sat down, quickly pulling off my Oakley trail-running shoes, then ripped my pants off. Otherwise still in full gear. I walked back to my room at the compound pant-less, head hanging, rifle slung across my chest, in full body armor. *Why does this keep happening to me?!*

I supposed I could have opted out for this mission, seeing as how sick I was, but I couldn't bear missing the action and fighting alongside my brothers. I was suffering because I'd chosen to do so.

✪

With our struggles and accomplishments come the problems we ultimately choose to take on. It all goes back to the choices we make. Even when we make good choices, we set ourselves up for new problems—they are just better than the problems that would have come with bad choices. Do we avoid life's many problems and challenges when we stay safely in our comfort zone? Sure, maybe. Can we avoid making bad choices when we don't take any risk? Yes. But what potential bad problems could arise within the confines of our comfort zone? Depression? Dissatisfaction? Mediocrity? Always asking yourself, "What if?" All the above?

Would anyone admit they are satisfied with the status quo? That mediocrity is just fine by them? Actually, yes. Some people would. But they are fooling themselves. Comfort zone expansion is a pathway to finding new opportunities that could never be seized without a little bit of calculated risk. My ultimate decision to quit my new job and join the Navy went over like a turd in a punch bowl among close friends and family. Picture that.

You're going to do what? Have you lost your mind?

Brent, that's a huge risk. You have to join the Navy first, then attempt to be accepted into the program. Then you have to actually make it through—and most people don't! Then you'll just be stuck in the Navy.

Oh, and isn't it like really dangerous?

All valid points.

My decision didn't come overnight, of course. It was a long process of training and weighing risk. But I knew the harder I trained and prepared, the lower the risk could potentially be. I say "potentially" because there are just too many unseen obstacles. Failure. Quitting. Being dropped for underperformance. Severe injury. Death. But I knew that deciding not to take on this challenge would lead to bad problems. Regret. Depression. Mediocrity. Always asking, "What if?"

Naturally, my decision to leap over the wall of my comfort zone and race off into the abyss would come with new problems. New struggles. New pain. These would prove, however, to be good problems. Problems I essentially chose by taking the road less traveled.

I forced myself to suffer in the mountains of Colorado for months before joining the Navy. We experienced extreme suffering during Hell Week and the pain of losing a brother. Each day at dusk, the instructors lined us up on the beach and made us wave goodbye to the sun as it slowly melted into the horizon—a ritual for welcoming the bitter cold and darkness soon to follow. Nights that seemed like they would never end. Yet each morning, the sun would rise again, warming our souls and saying, "You're one day closer to the end—keep going." We earned our Trident pins and soon discovered that life as a SEAL at war is full of sacrifice. Later, we suffered on the battlefield as we cut our teeth as wartime SEALs. But this was suffering we welcomed, as do the new warriors taking our place. We suffer at the loss of our sisters and brothers who sacrifice their lives for the teammates to their right and left. But if they were here today and you asked them if they had any regrets, they'd say, "Not one." Do they wish they'd made a different choice? Nope.

✪

Life is a series of choices. But how many choices do we make each day? How many are consequential? How many don't really matter? Some sources suggest that the average person makes up to 35,000 choices per day. Assuming that most people spend around seven hours per day sleeping and thus blissfully choice-free, that makes roughly 2,000 decisions per hour or one decision every two seconds. But does this enormous figure really hold up? Did some poor research assistant spend a whole day taking note of every minute detail of every fleeting choice that crossed her mind? Furthermore, any estimate will heavily depend on a person's very own definition of decision-making. Finally, not all decisions may be important in the grander scheme of things.

Whatever the statistics are, we cannot deny being faced with a never-ending stream of decisions from the moment we crawl out of bed in the morning. Sometimes, seemingly small choices can have monumental consequences. We must not underestimate the *butterfly effect*. Commonly cited in chaos theory, the butterfly effect is the idea that a small change can result in much more significant events—one tiny incident can have a huge impact on the future. By ignoring email or other notifications on your phone (which we should all do more of, frankly), you may miss an offer for your dream job or a one in a million match on a dating app. But then again, maybe it wasn't meant to be. Consider the decisions made on the field of battle. Every single choice you make has a consequence.

> *We're taking enemy fire from an elevated position. Do we engage or retreat? Call air support or not?*
>
> *I've been staring at an enemy target through a scope for three hours. Do I close my eyes for a minute and risk missing the crucial shot? What would the consequences be?*
>
> *An enemy combatant is acting violent and hostile but doesn't appear to have a weapon? What about a suicide vest? Do I engage? If I'm wrong, will I be prosecuted for murder? What's the risk?*
>
> *Enemy squirters flee into a field. Do we pursue?*

Obviously, not everyone is faced with these types of choices that have life or death consequences. And I'm not suggesting we obsess over every single decision we make at work, at home, or at Starbucks. Instead, I am arguing for more awareness of the vast quantity of choices that present themselves each day. Decisions large and small.

No matter the exact number of daily decisions we make, we might as well pay attention to them, because—as author John C. Maxwell famously put it—"Life is a matter of choices, and every choice you make makes you."

The Village of Choice

Let's say you live in a small, sustainable, peaceful village. And that village is in the middle of a clearing, surrounded by a dense forest. The general consensus among your fellow villagers is that bad things live in the forest—scary beasts, thieves, venomous snakes, quicksand, tax collectors, the potential for starvation, and, of course, rodents of unusual size. Under no circumstances do you go into the forest.

But what's really out there? Nobody knows because no brave soul has ventured beyond the borders of the safe and peaceful village. The villagers have convinced themselves that they are happy. Some of them truly are, because they don't know any better. But you? You're bored out of your fucking mind. You're curious. You have a fire burning deep inside, a voice asking, *What if?*

So, one day you say, "Screw it." Maybe there are scary things lurking out there. Maybe there is the possibility for pain, even death. But maybe there are great things beyond boring village life. Who the hell wants to farm squash and tend to pigs their whole life, only to end up marrying their cousin? Not you. Hell no. So you go for it. You pack a small bag with a few necessary items and head out.

Later that night you make camp and start a small fire to keep warm. You soon realize it's pretty cold out there at night. And dark. Boy, is it dark. And a bit scary. You keep hearing weird sounds. Possibly the scary beasts or tax collectors?

As you drift off into a restless sleep, your mind wanders back to your cozy little hut back in the village. It's warm, and there is a pot of squash stew on the stove and lanterns casting a gentle glow across the room. It sure would be nice to be tucked into your bed rather than curled up, shivering on a mossy boulder.

The next morning you awake, alive and well. You haven't been eaten alive by a beast or bitten by a poisonous snake. You're actually comfortable being a little uncomfortable because you chose to venture out. You're satisfied with your decision because now you know a bit more about what's out there. You pack up and head deeper into the forest. Ten minutes later, you twist your ankle on a slippery log and get attacked by a swarm of oddly aggressive mosquitos. You then remember that a friend once told you that mosquitos kill more people every year than any other predator—something about malaria. You're screwed. But you keep moving forward—and you don't die.

When you're in hell, just keep going.

—WINSTON CHURCHILL

You remind yourself that these are good problems and some suffering you'd rather have than, say, depression, boredom, and mediocrity. You can now proudly claim the title of adventurer! Later that afternoon you come to a clearing. You step out of the dense forest into what happens to be a thriving metropolis. There are beautiful buildings, and happy, gorgeous people are bustling down the avenues, clearly on their way home from amazing jobs they adore (probably not farming squash) and into the arms of loved ones they deeply care for. It's clearly paradise—a utopia you would never have known about if you didn't leave. You decide right then and there that you'll never go back to the village. Sure, it took a little bit of suffering to get there (not as much as you thought), but now you can get the medical attention you need and find amazing new opportunities.

Many people prefer to stay in their comfortable village. If they do venture out, it's not very far. People stay in jobs they hate because they are too fearful of the risk involved in quitting and finding something new. They stay in unfulfilling relationships for years, only to be consumed by regret and the feeling that they've wasted their life. We postpone tough decisions we know need to be made because the idea of confrontation gives us deep anxiety. People quickly adopt a victim mindset because things never seem to go their way. They aren't as lucky as all those successful and "happy" people they see on social media. They don't ask for that promotion they know they deserve due to fear of rejection.

These are all choices. Bad choices, indecision, and inaction lead to bad problems. Good decisions, calculated risk, and action lead to good problems. Which do you prefer? Why not choose what you are willing to suffer for rather than letting life—or others—choose for you?

✪

SERE school sucks. Advanced SERE is even worse. SERE (Survival, Evasion, Resistance, Escape) school is a program for teaching special operators and fighter pilots how to evade the enemy and withstand the suffering of being a POW.

It was a cold, dark night in an undisclosed location in California. I was three months away from deploying to Iraq for my first combat deployment. A few of my platoon mates and I had been sent to SERE. SEALs can't deploy to a combat zone without having taken the course. The instructors were all speaking Russian and never broke character.

I was starting to forget that this was just training. In the mock POW camp, my home was a small cement cubbyhole just large enough for the fetal position. I had spent the previous five days navigating the deep woods with an Air Force fighter pilot attempting to evade the enemy. Each night we'd spoon under a bush trying to share body heat. They only allow you to carry ChapStick and water. No food. By the fourth day, I had eaten both of my sticks of strawberry ChapStick. It tasted better than a meal at a five-star restaurant. It was awesome.

I was standing against a cement wall in one of the interrogation rooms. I had been dragged from my tiny cell where I'd laid shivering in my underwear all night, dreaming about what I would eat when I got home. The bright spotlight pointed at my face was blinding, but its warmth was a welcome change from the thirty-five degree December air temperature.

Two of my muscle-bound "captors" stood to my right and left. An interrogator was seated at the desk in front of me. I was desperately trying to recall the week of classroom training we'd had prior to being flung into the wilderness.

The questioning began. I attempted to use the techniques I learned in class. *I'm so tired. I don't remember much. I think I'm injured. Name. Rank. Serial number. Stick to your story. Lie without actually lying.* My captors weren't convinced. SMACK! A huge paw slammed against my face, flipping my head 90 degrees to the right. *What the fuck?* Blood trickled down my chin. Now I was pissed. SMACK! The other man's meaty hand came from the opposite direction. My blood was boiling, and I desperately tried to control my emotions. I didn't do a good job. I lunged at one of the instructors with a flurry of well-intentioned curse words as my only weapon. The other instructor was on me in a millisecond; he put me in an impressive chokehold.

The instructor playing the role of interrogator stood quickly and broke character, calling a brief training time-out. "Gleeson, you pull shit like that again and we'll just fail you," he said in a calm, professional tone. Basically, I had to sit there and take it. You know, get the full benefit and training value. Otherwise, I'd fail and not be able to deploy. Then, the training time-out was over, and it was back to the old slap and tickle. Then a bucket of water and some rags were brought into the room. I'll let your imagination take it from there.

★

Sometimes embracing the suck ... well ... sucks! And we don't always choose our suffering. Why do innocent people suffer injustice, racism, and inequality? Why does a parent have to die and leave young children, or why does a person have to lose a leg, their ability to move, or their eyesight? Why does a person have to suffer from rape or cancer, or get killed in combat? For some, the greatest pain may be not knowing why they suffer. Suffering is often easier to bear when we understand its purpose. When we are able to accept it and shift focus toward the potentially positive aspects of our existence.

And then there is purposeful suffering. The kind of suffering that is necessary to become truly fulfilled. Psychologists have studied the area of happiness extensively and the findings are what most assume, but few of us are willing to accept. The more things we acquire, money we make, or recognition we receive for accomplishing great—but sometimes meaningless—goals, our happiness level actually decreases. But when we strip away the material items or push the limits of our comfort zone, our happiness increases. Why? Because our perspective on what matters to us changes.

I guarantee that training for—and competing in—a challenging race would bring you more happiness and fulfillment than buying a new car. Investing your limited time to give back or support a cause close to your heart will always bring more joy than yet another social engagement with friends you see all the time. Being disciplined about your fitness and wellness routine would bring you far greater satisfaction than making a little more money every year. A BUD/S student's morale during Hell Week soars just by putting on dry socks, even though the rest of him is soaking wet and chilled to the bone.

The term "perception is reality" usually has a bit of a negative connotation. But it doesn't have to. If we change our perception of adversity, imagine what could be possible. As British Explorer Sir Ernest Shackleton once said, "Difficulties are just things to overcome, after all." Simple right? If we all could embrace that mindset, life's challenges wouldn't seem so bad. But Ernest was a bit of a different breed.

He was a British polar explorer who led three expeditions to the Antarctic, and one of the principal figures of the period known as the Heroic Age of Antarctic Exploration. During the second expedition (1907–1909) he and three companions established a new record by making the largest advance toward the South Pole in exploration history. For this achievement, Ernest was knighted by King Edward VII upon his return home.

After the race to the South Pole ended in December 1911, he turned his attention to the crossing of Antarctica from sea to sea, via the pole. To this end, he made preparations for what became the Imperial Trans-Antarctic Expedition, which lasted for three grueling years. Ernest published details of his new expedition early in 1914. Two ships would be employed; *Endurance* would carry the main party into the Weddell Sea, aiming for Vahsel Bay. From there, a team of six, led by Ernest, would begin the crossing of the continent. Meanwhile, a second ship, the *Aurora*, would take a supporting party under Captain Aeneas Mackintosh to McMurdo Sound on the opposite side of the continent. This party would then lay supply depots across the Great Ice Barrier as far as the Beardmore Glacier. These depots would be stocked with the food and fuel that would enable Ernest's party to complete their journey of 1,800 miles across the continent. Sounds super fun, right?

Legend has it that Ernest posted this ad in the *Times* when recruiting for the expedition. It read:

> *Men wanted for hazardous journey. Low wages, bitter cold, long hours of complete darkness. Safe return doubtful. Honor and recognition in event of success.*

Sounds like a Navy SEAL recruiting poster! Ours might read:

> *Low pay. More misery than you could imagine. Potential for death. But hey, you get to be a pipe hitter, serve your country, and purge the world of evil. —Uncle Sam*

I know what you're thinking. *Well that sure was stupid. Ernest clearly was no marketing expert. Definitely not a talent acquisition professional. Good luck with that!* Actually, over the coming weeks, 5,000 crazy bastards applied for the expedition. These people were clearly nuts! Maybe they all thought the ad was a joke, but it was no joke. Basically, the applicants were saying, "I'll take an order of pain and suffering with a side of misery and potential death please." But with the promise of adventure and possible noteworthy achievement, that was enough.

As usual, Murphy came a-callin'. Disaster struck this expedition when *Endurance* became trapped in pack ice and was slowly crushed before the shore parties could be delivered to land. The crew escaped by camping on the sea ice for many miserable months, living off limited rations supplemented by raw seal and dog meat. No ChapStick, apparently. Embrace the suck, gents—you signed up for it! Shackleton's recruiting ad was accurate after all.

Eventually, the ice disintegrated enough for them to launch the lifeboats and reach Elephant Island. Ultimately, they inhabited the island of South Georgia, after a stormy ocean voyage of 720 nautical miles. It was Ernest's most famous exploit. In 1921, he returned to the Antarctic, but died of a heart attack while his ship was moored in South Georgia. He was buried there at his wife's request.

Sir Ernest Shackleton was a man driven by ambition. Away from his expeditions, his life was generally restless and unfulfilled. In his search for rapid pathways to wealth and security, he launched business ventures that failed to prosper, and he died heavily in debt. Upon his death, he was lauded in the press, but was thereafter largely forgotten. But later in the twentieth century, he was rediscovered and rapidly became a role model for leadership as someone who, in extreme circumstances, kept his team together.

One could argue that at his core he may have been driven by the wrong values, as we discussed in Chapter Three, but he clearly had a drive that fueled his ability to achieve lofty goals. That same drive (fire) ended up saving the lives of his crew. His career was full of extreme suffering that he specifically chose in pursuit of his passions.

Mental Model

Suffering Practices

In the early days of my entrepreneurial adventures, I felt a lot like Sir Ernest. Adrift in uncharted waters. Running low on supplies. Safe return on investment doubtful. Occasionally gnawing on raw seal meat. I'll admit, it was very challenging and stressful. But it was also extremely fulfilling, because it was mine to own. It was suffering I chose once again. As I mentioned, start-ups have a similar failure rate as SEAL training, but I didn't care. Because I'd already pushed the boundaries of my comfort zone beyond what I could have ever imagined, I knew that this path could be successful as well. Not without obstacles, anxiety, and failure, but ultimately successful.

So, it's not just about being more thoughtful in choosing what you are willing to suffer for, but also *how* to engage in proper suffering. Almost every self-help book seems to be about how to be happy, how to be empowered and engage in positive self-talk, how to be in a fabulous relationship, how to build wealth . . . in other words, how to be anything other than the inevitably suffering human beings most of us are at some point in our lives. But we all experience suffering, so why fight it? Better to embrace it, understand it, and learn to walk the path in harmony. Better to understand the steps we take to arrive at suffering and learn how to navigate these trying periods in our lives in a more healthy manner.

The Embrace the Suck model has five suffering practices that are backed by research to help you grow through times of struggle.

1. Find safe relationships to process suffering. Suffering is meant to be dealt with in a relationship. We all need people to walk alongside us on the journey of suffering. We know from research and experience that social support plays a huge role in helping people cope with trials and eventually grow from them. You need people who provide a safe place for you to express your true feelings about your pain. Even though it's difficult when you're going through a hard time, you need to do your part in reaching out and being vulnerable. A deeper appreciation of vulnerability is one of the positive changes people tend to experience when they grow through suffering.

2. Face and express your emotions. Once you find people to walk with you on this journey, you need to approach and express your emotions, rather than suppress and run from them. It's commonly known that sharing your emotions related to suffering leads to positive outcomes. Conversely, research indicates that suppressing emotions leads to negative outcomes, like increased rates of anxiety and depression. You need emotionally safe relationships in order to do this. You have to trust that your vulnerable emotions will be handled with care and compassion. When you express your true emotions in the context of safe relationships, it sets in motion a series of positive processes. You connect more deeply to others, which is healing in itself. In addition, you begin to discover the meaning of your suffering in the context of your life story.

3. Process the emotions of suffering all the way through. Once you start talking about and feeling the pain of your suffering, stay with the feelings until you get to the end of the emotional arc. This principle comes from what is sometimes called a functional theory of emotion, which suggests that emotions are fundamentally adaptive. Emotions are your automatic evaluation of the events in your life. They provide information that is crucial, and they orient you to what is important for your well-being. For example, sadness is adaptive because it helps you grieve a loss. Emotions have a natural arc, or progression, in terms of their intensity and clarity. As you begin to feel the impact of your trial, you may start off ruminating about the situation. It's important that you don't stop at this phase. You need to embrace your emotions more fully to experience their adaptive benefits. As you engage in this process with people you trust and continue the arc of the feeling, the meaning becomes clearer, and there is a sense of relief as you experience the full measure of your own emotional truth.

4. Reflect on and reorder your priorities. Trials have a way of making you rethink your priorities in life. This can help you grow. But you must actively reflect on what is truly important to you and then be intentional about changing your routines, habits, and rhythms in ways that align with your revised priorities. That might mean spending more time with your spouse and kids and cherishing each present moment with them. It could mean accepting and even embracing your limitations. Maybe it's leaving the next item on your to-do list undone when the time has come to do something else, and trusting that you will complete the work in order of priority. Or possibly it means finding your identity through relationships rather than accomplishments.

5. Use your experiences of suffering to help others. Many people find an immense sense of meaning in helping others who've gone through similar trials. Even if others didn't experience the same challenges as you, using your pain as the fuel for empathy and compassion for others is a way of redeeming your suffering. It helps you create meaning out of it. Many veterans suffering from PTSD find peace in serving fellow veterans. Research shows that volunteerism is one of the most powerful ways we can engage in our own healing. In the same way, this is a core reason grieving parents of fallen soldiers start foundations in their name. And frankly, that's why I serve as a board member for the SEAL Family Foundation as well as mentor young men into and through the SEAL training program. So, get off your ass and go find a cause greater than yourself. Trust me, you'll never regret it.

Great, So What Now?

So, whether the pain and emotional obstacles we experience are chosen or dealt to us, practicing purposeful suffering undoubtedly leads to a better life. BUD/S students who make it through training can bear the suffering—lean into it even—because they have chosen to accept it as a means to a better end. A pathway to a specific goal. It's no different for elite athletes, successful entrepreneurs, or anyone who has chosen to expand their comfort zone in pursuit of something they are passionate about. It's a willingness we all have if we just tap into it. If you just embrace the suck and the good problems that will undoubtedly follow, you'll eventually find greatness—whatever your definition of that is.

Challenge yourself to identify both the suffering you have chosen, the suffering you haven't, and the meaning in it all. Consider how you can derive positive benefits from your most arduous and painful times. What perspective could be gained and applied to transforming your mind?

Questions to ask yourself:

What problems can I identify in my life currently? In the past? Did they stem from good choices or bad choices?

Do I embrace the challenges I face when pursuing aggressive goals and new opportunities, or do I allow those obstacles to turn me around—to push me back in the direction of my safe village?

What potential satisfaction could I derive from taking more risk in life?

What do I willingly suffer for and why?

Do I have the ability to change my perspective on the suffering I didn't choose?

What potentially amazing things could I discover about myself by engaging in purposeful suffering?

PART 3

TAKE ACTION: EXECUTE, EXECUTE, EXECUTE

In the absence of orders, I will take charge.

—NAVY SEAL ETHOS

8

WIN MORE THROUGH DISCIPLINE AND ACCOUNTABILITY

The first and best victory is to conquer self.

—PLATO

I n the early stages of BUD/S, all students are divided into boat crews, seven-person teams that consist of six enlisted students and one officer, the boat crew leader. This teaches prospective SEALs to work diligently in small teams just like on the battle-field and requires teamwork, communication, discipline, and accountability—all paramount skills for team success in any environment. Team discipline and accountability begins and ends with *personal* discipline and accountability and demands total engagement from each team member. The crews that win the most have members who look out for the person to their left and right more than themselves, which creates an overlapping web of high performance.

We demand discipline. We expect innovation.

—NAVY SEAL ETHOS

During Hell Week, many of the activities involve competition with the other crews. Some crews come together quickly; they are highly disciplined and work collaboratively to achieve their goals. Each team member holds themselves and the others to the highest standard. When they fall short, they debrief and apply lessons learned for continuous improvement. *Kaizen* is Japanese for resisting the plateau of arrested development—otherwise, never being satisfied with the status quo. Its literal translation is "continuous improvement." These crews find strength in one another during the most arduous times. The leaders inspire the team by taking on the hardest tasks and carrying more than their share of the weight. And they win, consistently. Other crews succumb to the pain, suffering, and misery and fall apart. They allow external influences to deteriorate their personal and team-level accountability and discipline. Infighting and finger-pointing ensues. And they lose, consistently.

Sometimes the instructors perform what I refer to as leadership experiments. They take the leader from the crew that is consistently winning all or the majority of the races and swap them out with the leader of the crew that is losing the majority of the races, then sit back and see what unfolds. The outcome is relatively consistent across classes and quite fascinating. The crew that was always dragging in the rear, under new inspirational leadership, almost immediately moves to the middle or near the head of the pack. Why? Because the leader knows how to quickly transform the mindsets of the individuals and culture of the team. To reignite their aggression. To give them that collective passion—a will to win as a team through discipline and accountability. They become inspired, and unified, and they operate under a new mission narrative they can emotionally connect to.

Meanwhile, the crew that was winning the majority of the races, under new seemingly poor leadership, continues to lead the pack! Why? Because the winning culture and mindset of each team member was already so ingrained that no one person or externality could dismantle what they'd created. The level of individual and team discipline they have forged is unbreakable, even in the worst of conditions. They thrive on adversity.

In BUD/S, SQT, and selection programs for other elite NSW special mission units, the instructors weigh data from peer reviews heavily. On a regular basis, the members of the class anonymously rank their peers with the opportunity to provide explanations. If you have ever done a 360-degree review in your company, you get the idea. So, imagine a 360-degree review on steroids where the stakes are extremely high. Students who are consistently ranked at the bottom are brought in for a board review and considered for removal. But the reasoning for a candidate being rated poorly by their classmates may not be what you imagine. It's not because they aren't the fastest runner, the best swimmer, or a proficient shooter on the range. It's behavioral. The student lacks discipline, integrity, and accountability. They don't put the team's needs before their own. They fear failure and therefore don't take calculated risks. They lack creativity and innovation. Basically, they are someone you wouldn't want to be standing next to in a gunfight in Ramadi.

Discipline and accountability aren't just the path to winning more in your life, but the true gateway to happiness and fulfillment. Think about it this way. I'm sure you've come across people in your life who seem to always put in the required work and effort for any given task, be it their job, a hobby, or maybe a fitness goal. Yet the result or outcome seems to be consistently lackluster. Then others who put in the same amount of time and perceived effort seem to always be in a state of kaizen—continuous improvement. If both groups are putting in the time, why would the result be different? Research on this topic brought me to K. Anders Ericsson, a Swedish psychologist and Conradi eminent scholar and professor of psychology at Florida State University, who is internationally recognized in the field of human performance and expertise.

In their *Harvard Business Review* article, "The Making of an Expert," Ericsson, Michael J. Prietula, and Edward T. Cokely provide deep insight into the subject of *deliberate practice*. They argue that it's not so much about the time invested, but rather how we go about pursuing continuous improvement. I didn't become a proficient open water swimmer by floating in the Pacific for hours on end. You don't become a great golfer simply by hitting the course three days a week with your buddies—especially if you're slamming Busch Light tallboys the whole time. I'd imagine even the top hotdog eating champions have worked deliberately on their craft.

In the beginning of the article, they highlight the work of Benjamin Bloom, a professor of education at the University of

Chicago who published a revolutionary book called *Developing Talent in Young People,* which examined the critical factors that contribute to talent. Bloom's studies focused on what sets apart effort from developing true expertise. His work focused on musicians, artists, mathematicians, and athletes. Three key areas he highlights as differentiators are:

1. Intense and focused practice
2. Study with devoted teachers
3. Support from family during key developmental years

A quote from the article that can't be overlooked is this:

The journey to truly superior performance is neither for the faint of heart nor for the impatient. The development of genuine expertise requires *struggle, sacrifice,* and honest, often *painful self-assessment.* There are no shortcuts. It will take you at least a decade to achieve expertise, and you will need to invest that time wisely, by engaging in "deliberate" practice—practice that focuses on tasks *beyond your current level of competence and comfort.* Moving beyond your traditional comfort zone of achievement requires substantial motivation and sacrifice, but it's a necessary discipline.

We train for war and fight to win.

—NAVY SEAL ETHOS

To illustrate this point, one of the most critical and unfortunately relevant skills SEALs must master is close quarters combat (CQC). Much of the fighting we have done over the past two decades has been in urban environments—large cities and dense rural villages—which is arguably the most dangerous type of combat due to 360 degrees of threats. CQC training is predominantly performed in a structure called a *kill house*. One of our famous training mottos is "slow is smooth and smooth is fast." Basically, the crawl-walk-run philosophy. You begin learning the trade in BUD/S and then start refining your skills in SQT. Safety violations in the kill house are one of the fastest ways to get dropped from training due to the extremely serious nature of this craft. We train in live-fire scenarios. Yes, real bullets in tight spaces. The goal is to capture or eliminate enemy threats without putting a round through your teammate's head or shooting an undeserving noncombatant.

In the kill house, well-trained SEAL instructors watch your every move from a web of catwalks that span the entire structure. One evolution might be that the team will breach an exterior door, then dynamically enter the house moving down corridors clearing room by room. Each room has a different scenario set up; armed combatants mixed with noncombatants, hostage situations, different furniture configurations, you name it. Instructors who hold your future in their hands watch every move in extreme detail. Body position, foot movement, appropriate speed, muzzle discipline, following best practices, everything. Oh, and don't shoot the fucking hostage! That will earn you some serious remediation. The kill house we use at Marine Corps Base Camp Pendleton, for example, has a ridiculously steep hill next to it—a small mountain, really. If you throw a round off target, shoot the hostage, or incur a safety violation, your ass runs the hill in full gear.

All of our training is deliberate, and as the SEAL Ethos says, "My training is never complete." Being in a constant state of kaizen is critical for our survival. Painful self-assessment (and peer feedback) is our prescription for enhanced performance. This continuum expands your comfort zone to the farthest reaches you could ever imagine. We train deliberately. Assess performance. Then train again.

Team Accountability

As previously alluded to, personal discipline and accountability directly apply to success in a team setting as well. In my first book, *TakingPoint: A Navy SEAL's 10 Fail-Safe Principles for Leading Through Change*, I argue that accountability is the most critical cultural pillar for high performance in any team environment, especially as it relates to navigating the murky waters of volatility and uncertainty—a battlefield the whole world is now accustomed to.

Consider the following story of Dave Schlotterbeck, formerly the CEO of Alaris Medical Systems. It's a case study of a leader who learned to master change in his organization and bring impressive results to the bottom line by building a culture that embraces total accountability. And while his organization wasn't being bombarded by a global pandemic, attacked by a swarm of hungry locusts, or threatened with death and dismemberment, its journey from the depths is proof that accountability is the road to true transformation, whether it be personal or professional, team or individual. Dave knew that he needed to change the organizational culture at Alaris. People were avoiding risks and shrinking from opportunities out of fear of failure, and there was a total lack of discipline. Like BUD/S boat crews that consistently lose the race. Almost everyone in the organization was more worried about protecting themselves and finding another job than getting the results the company needed. Dave recognized that to change the results, he would need to change the mindset, how people interacted, and the way they approached their work—the culture. So he went in search of a new approach to transform the organization. I refer to this as a "culture-driven transformation."

Dave led the process for redefining the company's rituals and beliefs so they better aligned with the actions necessary to achieve desired results. He transformed the Alaris culture and literally changed the landscape of the medical systems industry. In just three years, Alaris increased its share price from $.31 per share to $22.35 per share, growing as much as 15 percent a year in a market where competitors were achieving no more than 3 percent. Soon thereafter, the company was acquired by Cardinal Health, a Fortune 20 company, and later spun out as the nucleus of CareFusion—one of TakingPoint Leadership's clients. Today, CareFusion is one of the largest medical device suppliers in the world. Dave describes the culture change at Alaris as the "most difficult job" he had to perform during his distinguished forty-year career, but it's also the one he takes greatest pride in. Why? Because it was so fucking uncomfortable—my words, not his. Learning how to change a culture, and change it quickly, is a vital part of the new leadership skill set required for operating in volatile, uncertain, complex, and ambiguous environments, whether it's business, family, relationships, or the battlefield.

Based on that story, consider how discipline and accountability not only apply in a team setting but also to our own personal and professional performance.

✪

When I was in middle school, I fell in love with rock climbing. I enjoyed the physical and mental challenge of it, and actually discovered I enjoy heights. My twin brother and I attended a hardcore expedition camp each summer that involved rock climbing, ice climbing, and mountaineering. By the time we finished high school, we'd become relatively proficient climbers and had summited several of the highest peaks in North America. My twin was far more advanced than I was, however. From the ice-covered peaks of Wind River in Wyoming to the jungles of Costa Rica, there was definitely some purposeful, blissful suffering that came in handy later in my career as a SEAL.

Those with a passion for climbing aren't all cut from the same cloth. And some are purely insane. Take Alex Honnold, for example. He's a master of focus and discipline in his trade. Alex lived in a van in Yosemite National Park for over a decade. No, he wasn't homeless— he just wanted to live in a van and climb all day, every day. He is best known for his free solo ascents of big rock walls. How big? Insanely big. And what do I mean by free solo? I mean not using any ropes.

Alex is the author (with David Roberts) of the memoir *Alone on the Wall* and the subject of the 2018 biographical documentary *Free Solo*. As one of his close climbing friends and colleagues said in an interview in the documentary, "Imagine an event in the Olympics, but if you don't earn the gold medal, you die."

Alex was born in Sacramento, California. He started climbing in a gym at the age of five. By age ten he was climbing every day and he participated in many national and international youth climbing championships as a teenager. He had found a passion, and he was extremely disciplined in his quest to fulfill that passion. His practice was *deliberate*.

In a *Rolling Stone* interview he said, "I was never, like, a bad climber as a kid, but I was never a great climber, either. There were a lot of other climbers who were much, much stronger than me, who started as kids and were, like, instantly freakishly strong— like they just have a natural gift. And that was never me. I just loved climbing, and I've been climbing all the time ever since, so I've naturally gotten better at it, but I've never been gifted."

Okay, whatever you say, Alex. Whatever you say.

He gained mainstream recognition after his 2012 solo of the Regular Northwest Face of Half Dome and was featured in the film *Alone on the Wall* and a subsequent *60 Minutes* interview. In 2014, Clif Bar announced that it would no longer sponsor Alex, along with four other climbers, who were mostly free soloists. "We concluded that these forms of the sport are pushing boundaries and taking the element of risk to a place where we as a company are no longer willing to go," the company wrote in an open letter. Basically, saying: We can no longer support your lunacy and suicidal tendencies!

On June 3, 2017, he made the first ever free solo ascent of El Capitan, completing the 2,900-foot Freerider route in three hours and fifty-six minutes. The feat, described as one of the greatest athletic feats of any kind, ever, was documented by climber and photographer Jimmy Chin, and was the subject of the 2018 documentary. The good news is that the film didn't turn out to be a tragedy!

What makes him so good? The fact that he *really, really* gives a shit about climbing. In fact, it's one of the few things he really cares about. And that passion drives his discipline and accountability. And he uses his passion and talent to give back. The Honnold Foundation is a nonprofit organization dedicated to bringing solar energy to impoverished communities. Alex not only uses his fame and connections to support this goal, but he also donates a whopping one-third of his income to the foundation every year.

> Interestingly, research supports the fact that when our passions can lead to giving to causes greater than ourselves, we are more successful and dramatically more fulfilled.

We only have so many things we can really give a shit about in this short life. If we try to give a shit about everything, chase every shiny object that passes us, or have too many goals, we end up with mediocrity. Multitasking simply means you're doing many things in a half-assed, distracted manner all at once. We have to pick something. We must prioritize in order to execute. For Alex, it's climbing. For David Goggins, it's running and other ridiculously painful endeavors. For Sir Ernest, it was exploration. For Louis, it was purely survival. For me, it's dating my wife. Did I write that to score some points? Damn right I did.

Happiness and fulfillment come from focus, discipline, and self-control. It may be hard to believe when you're facing an all-you-can-eat buffet, the prospect of making a quick buck, or the lazy lure of sleeping in versus getting on the Peloton, but studies show that people with self-discipline are happier. Why? Because with discipline and self-control we actually accomplish more of the goals we truly care about.

> You have power over your mind—not outside events. Realize this, and you will find strength.
>
> —MARCUS AURELIUS

People with a higher degree of self-control spend less time debating whether to indulge in behaviors and activities that don't align with their values or goals. They are more decisive. They don't let impulses or feelings dictate their choices. Instead, they make levelheaded choices—even if those decisions involve some calculated risk. They are the architects of their own beliefs and the actions they take to achieve a desired outcome. As a result, they aren't as easily distracted by Temptation Tiger and tend to feel more satisfied with their lives.

Mental Model

Mastering Self-Discipline

There are actions you can take to learn self-discipline and gain the willpower to live a happier, more fulfilling life. If you are looking to take control of your habits and choices, here are the nine most powerful things you can do to master self-discipline—which, again, is imperative for life beyond your comfort zone—and maybe even redefining "extraordinary."

STEP ONE: Know your weaknesses.

We all have weaknesses. Whether they're the desire for alcohol, tobacco, unhealthy food, obsession over social media, or the video game *Fortnite* (what the hell is with this game, by the way?!), they have a similar effect on us. Weaknesses don't just come in the form of areas where we lack self-control either. We all have our strong suits and the stuff we kind of suck at. For example, I don't care for having difficult conversations (as I mentioned earlier), lengthy paperwork that involves digging up old documents I never saved in the first place, holding my temper when someone is shooting at me, picking up dog poop, or calling into automated phone systems. And therefore, I actively (or purposefully) suck at these activities. So, I strive to tackle them head-on—or I delegate them to others. (Never forget about the subtle art of delegation!)

Self-awareness is a powerful tool for comfort zone expansion, but it requires constant focus and acknowledging your shortcomings, whatever they may be. I suffered from bad allergies and asthma growing up, and had terrible eyesight. Those were some significant weaknesses when considering becoming a SEAL. But so what? I trained hard to improve my lung function and used money I'd saved for LASIK eye surgery. Too often people either try to pretend their vulnerabilities don't exist or they succumb to them with a fixed mindset, throwing their hands up in defeat and saying, "Oh well." Own up to your flaws. You can't overcome them until you do. What did Jason do when the doctors at Bethesda went down the list of shit he'd never be able to do again? Exactly.

If you haven't been zipped up by a high-caliber machine gun, you have no excuse.

STEP TWO: Remove temptations.

Like the saying goes, "out of sight, out of mind." It may seem silly, but this phrase offers powerful advice. By simply removing the biggest temptations from your environment, you will greatly improve your self-discipline. Just tell Temptation Tiger thank you for the invite, but you'll pass on the evening of debauchery.

When I decided I was going to pursue the lofty goal of becoming a SEAL, everything had to change. If you want to eat healthier, toss the junk food in the trash. Want to drink less? Throw out the booze. If you want to improve your productivity at work, turn off social media notifications and silence your cell phone. Prioritize and execute. The fewer distractions you have, the more focused you will be on accomplishing your goals. Set yourself up for success by ditching bad influences.

STEP THREE: Set clear goals and have an execution plan.

If you hope to achieve greater degrees of self-discipline, you must have a clear vision of what you hope to accomplish, just like any goal. You must also have an understanding of what success means to you. After all, if you don't know where you are going, it's easy to lose your way or get sidetracked. Remember to prioritize. When we work with our corporate clients on strategic planning, execution, and organizational transformation, we remind them that having ten priorities translates to *no* priorities.

A clear plan outlines each step you must take to reach your goals. If you want to become an ultramarathon runner, *most* of us don't start with a 100-mile race. Crawl, walk, run. Create a mantra to keep yourself focused. Successful people use this technique to stay on track and establish a clear finish line. At TakingPoint Leadership, we call this a *guiding metaphor*, something you can visualize and connect to. For example, one client uses "Always charge the net" because he loves tennis and has a goal to be more aggressive in his role at the company. In the coming pages, I'll provide you a detailed model that can be used for just about any objective.

STEP FOUR: Practice daily diligence.

We aren't born with self-discipline; it's a learned behavior. And just like any other skill you want to master, it requires daily practice and repetition. It must become habitual. But the effort and focus that self-discipline requires can be draining.

As time passes, it can become more and more difficult to keep your willpower in check. The bigger the temptation or decision, the more challenging it can feel to tackle other tasks that also require self-control. So, work on building your self-discipline through daily diligence. This goes back to step three. In order to practice daily diligence, you must have a plan. Put it on your calendar, your to-do list, whatever works best for you. With practice, anyone can do something that sucks every day.

STEP FIVE: Create new habits by keeping it simple.

Acquiring self-discipline and working to instill a new habit can feel daunting at first, especially if you focus on the entire task at hand. To avoid feeling intimidated, keep it simple. Break your goal into small, doable steps. Instead of trying to change everything at once, focus on doing one thing consistently and master self-discipline with that goal in mind. As we say in the SEAL Teams, "Eat the elephant one bite at a time."

If you're trying to get in shape but don't exercise regularly (or ever), start by working out ten or fifteen minutes a day. If you're trying to achieve better sleep habits, start by going to bed thirty minutes earlier each night. If you want to eat healthier, change your grocery shopping habits and prep your lunch the night before to take with you in the morning. Take baby steps. Eventually, when you're ready, you can add more goals to your list.

STEP SIX: Change your perception about willpower.

If you believe you have a limited amount of willpower, you probably won't surpass those limits. We have covered how willpower can deplete over time, but what about changing that perception? The BUD/S student who believes they probably won't make it through training won't succeed. Why assume our will to win can only take us so far? When we embrace the mindset of unlimited willpower, we continue to grow, achieve more, and develop mental toughness. It's the same philosophy as setting "stretch" goals.

In short, our internal conceptions about willpower and self-control can determine how disciplined we are. If you can remove these subconscious obstacles and truly believe you can do it, then you will give yourself an extra boost of motivation toward making those goals a reality.

STEP SEVEN: Give yourself a backup plan.

In the SEAL Teams, we always have contingency plans. Psychologists use a technique to boost willpower called "implementation intention." That's when you give yourself a plan to deal with a potentially difficult situation you know you will likely face. To be clear, I am not referring to a backup plan under the auspices that you'll probably fail at Plan A. Let's say you aspire to become a trapeze expert, but say to yourself, "Well, I'm probably going to suck at this, so chances are I'll be sticking with miniature golf." That's a crappy backup plan wrapped in mediocrity. We are talking about contingencies for intentional course correction, not planning for failure. So be bold and keep moving forward.

Going in with a plan will help give you the mindset and self-control necessary for the situation. You will also save energy by not having to make a sudden decision based on your emotional state.

STEP EIGHT: Find trusted coaches or mentors.

The development of expertise requires coaches who are capable of giving constructive, even painful, feedback. Real experts are extremely motivated students who seek out such feedback. They're also skilled at understanding when and if a coach's advice doesn't work for them.

The elite performers I've known and worked with always knew what they were doing right while concentrating on what they were doing wrong. They deliberately picked unsentimental coaches who would challenge them and drive them to higher levels of performance. The best coaches also identify aspects of your performance that will need to be improved at your next level of skill and aid you in preparation.

STEP NINE: Forgive yourself and move forward.

Even with all our best intentions and well-laid plans, we sometimes fall short. It happens. You will have ups and downs, great successes and dismal failures. The key is to keep going. A very close SEAL buddy of mine has had a lifelong dream of not just serving in the SEAL Teams but also making it to our tier one special missions unit. He has every qualification this unit could possibly want, but for some reason they didn't select him on his first application attempt. Did he wallow in sorrow? Not for one second. He immediately developed a plan to take more college courses and train even harder, and he transferred teams for a better chance to get picked up next time. Easy day.

If you stumble, find the root cause and move on. Don't let yourself get wrapped up in guilt, anger, or frustration, because these emotions will only drag you further down and impede future progress. Learn from your missteps and forgive yourself. Then get your head back in the game and violently execute.

Great, So What Now?

Well, for starters, make the choice to be more fucking disciplined. Hold yourself more accountable! These are choices that only you can make. No one else.

Give yourself time to master discipline and accountability holistically and in a given field. Remember, a disciplined mind leads to disciplined thought and disciplined action. I've found, for example, that greater discipline and personal accountability with fitness gives way to enhanced focus and follow-through in my business leadership ability. Think about it this way, if you were to measure your self-discipline, where would you place yourself on a scale of one to ten? Be honest with yourself. Self-discipline is one of the cornerstones of achievement, not just the achievement of big goals, but also the carrying out of simple daily tasks and chores.

Without a certain degree of self-discipline, you act like a jelly-fish. You get carried away by external forces, the environment, the media, family, or colleagues, floating aimlessly at the whim of the tides. Possessing self-discipline means to hold the steering wheel of your life and to become a doer, instead of a drifter.

Questions to ask yourself:

When I make a promise, trivial or important, do I keep it?

How often do I change my mind after making a decision?

Do I get up in the morning intending to do something, only to postpone it for later, and when the day is over, it is still not done?

When a certain action, task, or chore is difficult and takes time to accomplish, do I go through with it, or quit after a while?

If my answers to the above questions place me on the low end of discipline and accountability, what the hell am I going to do about it?

9

MODELING MINDSET AND BEHAVIOR FOR VIOLENT EXECUTION

The path to success is to take massive,
determined actions.

—TONY ROBBINS

Somewhere Over Iraq
2:00 A.M.

Our four CH-47 Chinook helicopters flew low and fast over the barren desert, filled with two SEAL platoons and Polish special operators on our way to the target: a massive hydroelectric power plant and dam that had been seized by retreating Iraqi forces. Our mission was to assault, capture, and hold the plant until conventional US forces arrived. The intelligence regarding the size and makeup of the enemy force protecting the plant wasn't very detailed. According to the intel, however, their intent was to destroy the dam, resulting in mass power and electrical outages and flooding of the land below. Our mission was to ensure this didn't happen.

This was our first combat mission in Iraq, but we hadn't even deployed "in-country" yet. We were still staged at Ali Al Salem Air Base in Kuwait doing our turnover with SEAL Team Three when we were handed this mission. As the helicopter rope suspension techniques (HRST) master in my platoon, my initial job was to prepare the helicopters and supervise the fast rope insert onto the target. I was sitting on a tight coil of thick green nylon rope next to the open door of the helicopter, monitoring our progress toward the insert point. I shivered slightly from the cold gusts blasting through the bird. Even though it was about 70 degrees outside, the stark contrast to the daytime heat—which was well above 100 degrees—confused the mind and body. We had been in flight for about three hours and our legs were numb and our bodies were stiff. The night sky was clear and illuminated by a full moon, which made it easier for us to see the landscape below but also made our helos nicely silhouetted targets for the enemy. Hills, dunes, and palm groves dotted the land beneath us.

"Ten minutes out," came the call over our radios. Now we were all awake. Each man passed the signal—ten fingers—down the line and checked weapons, radios, and night vision goggles. Each man double-checked the gear of the man next to him. We all put on our thick welding gloves that protected our hands from the intense friction that came from sliding down the nylon rope.

"Five minutes." Now, we were all on our feet, getting ready for the exit, hearts beating a little faster. Intense focus permeated our minds, each man envisioning his mission responsibilities. We had been rehearsing relentlessly day and night for this mission. When our platoon and the Polish GROM unit (elite special forces warriors) were tasked with this mission, we had been given roughly two weeks to prepare. And we train for war and fight to win.

We'd used every resource at our disposal to develop the mission plan, rehearse, poke holes in the plan, and rehearse again. We planned and trained for every possible contingency. We would dirt dive every choreographed move. Every decision. Every possible blockage. We used satellite imagery of the plant to build a framework of the compound, from landing zones to every structure on the target. We started by defining the objective, and identifying threats and necessary resource needs, then we used that information along with the intel at hand to determine go/no-go criteria. From there we assigned every possible action needed to fulfill the objective—what, who, when.

The helo crew chief and platoon commander leaned out to confirm our target location. "One minute." Each man passed the signal, one index finger extended. Hearts hammering, our point man (Mark Owen, who later went on to become a tier one special missions unit team leader and number one *New York Times* best-selling author of *No Easy Day* and *No Hero*) and I grabbed the coiled fast rope, lifted it up, and got ready to throw it out. The plant was enormous, stretching out across the horizon in front of us. Even the intense buzzing from our helicopter's spinning rotors didn't drown out the noise of the rushing river below us. There was no way to know exactly what was facing us, but anybody who was in that building and the surrounding structures had no idea what they were in for either. We'd all trained for years for this moment. It was time for the training wheels to come off.

Twenty feet above our landing zone, the helo came to a steady hover, and I threw out the rope, adrenalin masking the strain of seventy pounds of gear strapped to my body. Every man down the line gave a thumbs-up. With one final fist bump, we were ready to go. In rapid succession, each SEAL launched himself with well-trained precision out into the black abyss, grabbing the thick rope and sliding quickly down into the tornado of swirling sand below. We were ready to take the fight to the enemy.

I would be the final man to exit. As the last guy in the stack cleared the door on his way down, I leaned out and grabbed the rope. As it always was in training, the noise was deafening, the rotor wash intimidating. But what a fucking rush. With both hands on the rope, I let my body weight carry me forward and quickly began my descent. A split second later . . . *BAM!* With a sudden and violent jolt, my rapid downward motion ended.

Shit! I immediately knew what had happened. Despite a year of training for this deployment and two weeks deliberately practicing for this very moment, old Murphy came a callin' as usual. Anything that can go wrong will go wrong. Let me back up really quickly so you get the picture. This was my first platoon as a SEAL, so I'm one of three *new guys*. And new guys get to carry the heavy shit. So in addition to my body armor, helmet, night vision goggles, small day pack, suppressed M4 rifle, Sig Sauer P226 9mm pistol, CamelBak full of water, rifle and pistol magazines, radio, and a few grenades, I was also carrying a thirty-pound fully gassed quickie saw on my back. I'd zip-tied it to an old rucksack frame so I could wear it like a backpack. Well, now that fucker was caught on the floor of the helo. My body was dangling twenty feet above the concrete landing, and my hands were gripping the rope as if my life depended on it, because it did. The river below raged on both sides of the helipad. I looked down and could see that the rotor wash had already ripped the chain-link fence surrounding the landing zone out of the concrete.

Well, I'm really embracing the suck now, I thought. The torture of BUD/S was looking pretty good right about now. As I was about to lose my grip, I looked back over my shoulder at the crew chief standing behind me. He knew just what to do. With one swift kick, he dislodged the saw from the floor of the helo and down I went in somewhat of a freefall, my hands doing little to slow my descent. I hit the deck hard, feet first, then onto my back. My spine crackled over the massive metal cutting saw. The inertia caused my rifle to swing up and smack me in the face, splitting my right eyebrow open two inches wide down to the bone. A river of blood streamed down my face, but I didn't realize it until later when a teammate said, "Dude, what the hell happened to you?!"

I prayed for the air that had been so violently ripped from my lungs to return. I quickly unfucked myself, got to my feet, and sprinted up the hill to catch up with my team. Luckily, I was only one small cog in this highly matrixed team. At the same time I was attempting unintentional suicide, we had snipers fast roping onto the roof of the main structure, a SEAL mobility unit landing desert patrol vehicles (DPVs—think dune buggies with 50 caliber machine guns) around the perimeter, and our Polish GROM brothers fast roping into their predetermined sectors. As the primary assault force, we stacked along the side wall of the main entrance, set charges, and blew the metal doors off their hinges. And into the breach we went.

Ultimately, we were successful in our mission. We cleared the giant power plant, capturing the enemy and eliminating threats as we went. The next day we searched miles of dark, wet tunnels that snaked beneath the massive property. We held the target for three days, then passed the torch to conventional forces. We took no casualties other than one of our Polish teammates who broke his ankle during the fast rope.

★

As nineteenth-century Prussian military commander Helmuth von Moltke put it, "No plan survives first contact with the enemy." A more modern take on it comes from world-famous boxing champ Mike Tyson: "Everybody has a plan until they get punched in the mouth." Damn right, Mike, damn right. The point is, the best-laid plans come under fire. There is no such thing as a perfect plan.

> A good plan, violently executed now, is better than a perfect plan next week.
>
> —GENERAL GEORGE PATTON

Preparation and execution beat planning all day long. But you still have to plan. We teach our consulting clients, many of whom are multibillion-dollar global organizations, the TakingPoint Leadership planning, execution, and debriefing model. Much of that model is derived from how we plan in the SEAL Teams. Proper planning and debriefing create an ideal rhythm of execution and a constant state of kaizen.

I might ask you, "When you set a goal, do you usually have a plan for achieving that goal?" Your answer most likely would be, "Sure, of course." But how well do we actually plan? Do we use the right approach? Want to become more resilient? Get in better shape? Earn a promotion at work? Start your own business? Find the love of your life? Raise children into healthy, kind, responsible young adults? Swim the English Channel? Break the Guinness record for holding your breath (it's twenty-two minutes, by the way)? Go to Wharton for your MBA? Become a Navy SEAL or Green Beret? Well, what's your plan?

As we all know, great plans have both long- and short-term elements. Personal and professional. Macro and micro. Strategic and tactical. So, whether you are planning to open a neighborhood coffee shop, be accepted into Juilliard, or climb Mount Everest, you gotta have a plan. Not just any plan. You need to use a specific framework. And let me just say, embracing the suck is a lot easier when you have a solid plan of attack.

So, since you asked, here it is. And yes, all this needs to be documented on paper, in a Google Doc, whatever, so long as you can refer to it regularly.

STEP ONE: Define the objective.

The objective must be concise, quantifiable, time bound, and support the *strategic imperative*. What's a strategic imperative, you ask? Basically, a strategic imperative is a longer-term goal supported by a series of objectives. Let's take a look at a few different styles for Objective Statements. Depending on what you're trying to accomplish, I prefer to use slightly different approaches with varying degrees of specificity.

When it's a personal fitness goal, for example, I like to be very specific. When training for a marathon, your objective statement might look something like this: *By June 1, 2021, I will run a marathon in under three hours following XYZ training regime on a weekly basis and completing at least two twenty-mile runs during the two months prior to the race.*

When we run planning workshops with our corporate clients, we often use the objectives and key results (OKR) methodology. In this case, objectives are memorable qualitative descriptions of what you want to achieve. Objectives should be short, inspirational, and engaging—something you (or a team) can emotionally connect to. An objective should motivate and challenge you. Key results are a set of metrics that measure your progress toward the objective. For each objective, you should have a set of two to five key results. More than that and you won't remember them. Here's an example for a business team:

OBJECTIVE: Create an Awesome Customer Experience
Key Results:

→ Improve Net Promoter Score from X to Y.

→ Increase Repurchase Rate from X to Y.

→ Maintain Customer Acquisition Cost Under Z.

Either approach works well. The idea is that your primary objective is clear, inspiring, and easy to remember.

STEP TWO: Identify threats and blockages.
Now that you have a clear, concise, quantifiable objective, you need to start thinking about what stands in your way. Opening that coffee shop you've always dreamed about? Well, list all the things that could throw a wrench into that plan. What's going to punch you in the face? Maybe the price per square foot for rent is a bit higher than you anticipated and could go up again next year. The location

is okay but not ideal. You're uncertain about customer traffic. Your budget is limited—if things don't take off in one year, you'll have to find an investor or close the doors. A global pandemic pops up. Uncertainty! This list could go on and on.

Once you have your list of potential threats, bucket them into things that are in your control and things that are not in your control. Put the items outside your control off to the side. Maintain situational awareness, but don't waste too much time or energy on them. Your focus needs to be on mitigating the threats that are in your control. Stay in your three-foot world.

STEP THREE: List needed resources.

Planning to capture a high value ISIS leader? Well, what resources do you need? Ground intel. A direct action assault force. Quick reaction force. A comms plan. Air support. Information on enemy movement in the region. Guns and shit. Whatever you think you need to accomplish the mission.

Keep in mind that some resources you need might be at your disposal and some may not be and must be sourced or acquired. Running that marathon? Proper shoes would help. Maybe a trainer who specializes in distance running. Regardless, specifically note the resources not immediately at your disposal because those will require specific time-bound "actions." We'll get to that in a second.

STEP FOUR: Determine go/no-go.

Based on the objective, threats, and resources needed to accomplish the mission, determine if the mission is achievable. Do not use this as an easy way out. This is simply a method for ensuring your objective is reasonable, even if it's a stretch goal.

For example, one of the no-go criteria we listed as a threat during the planning process for the mission I described earlier in this chapter was a sandstorm, a threat out of our control. Well, guess what. Two nights in a row, while we were literally on the tarmac in our helos getting ready to take off, the mission was canceled due to sandstorms. What a shock!

STEP FIVE: Apply lessons learned.

This is where you ask yourself, "Have I or anyone I know attempted this before?" If so, consider what went well, didn't go so well, and any insights you could apply to this current plan. If you've never run a marathon before, go find someone who has, such as a friend, coach, or mentor. If you tried to open the same coffee shop when you lived in Seattle but you had to close the doors after a year, what happened last time that you need to note in this new plan to open in Austin. Take into account the good, bad, and ugly. If you plan to kidnap that ISIS dude, what happened the last time you accomplished a similar mission?

The list doesn't have to be long. Only note the most relevant lessons learned that apply. Once you have the list, you may need to go back and adjust the objective statement or key results.

STEP SIX: Create an action plan.

The action plan is a list of all the time-bound items that must be executed in order to fulfill the objective. That might mean obtaining the resources not immediately at your disposal or executing on the key performance indicators (KPIs) and milestones that need to happen between now and when the objective is to be completed.

Here is where discipline and accountability come back into play. Each action must have a what, who, and when. Make three columns on your planning sheet. The *what* is, of course, the action itself. The *who* is the person responsible or accountable for making it happen. Depending on the objective, that may not always be you. If this is a quarterly project based on your annual strategic business plan, there may be four or five different people needed in the *who* category. *When* refers to the time-bound nature of the plan. Each action needs a due date.

STEP SEVEN: Assemble your Red Team.

Here comes the fun and often frustrating part of the planning process. Now that you have the plan about 60 percent complete—keeping in mind we are only taking it to 80 percent, which I'll explain in a minute—it's time to gain an outside perspective. And by perspective, I mean have two or three other people poke holes in your plan.

First, select a couple people with some relevant knowledge of you and your plan or goal. This is your *Red Team*. Next, present your plan: objective, threats, resources, go/no-go criteria, lessons learned, and associated actions. Allow them a few minutes to digest and ask clarifying questions if needed. For this to be done properly, the Red Team members will take turns saying only, "Have you considered . . . " Your *only* response is, "Thank you." No rebuttals, no arguments. So, for example, when you present your plan for running that marathon and your neighbor (an avid runner) says, "Have you considered that you're a lazy piece of shit who has never followed through with a fitness goal . . . ever?" After a brief, uncomfortable moment, your response is, "Thank you!" Jot down the relevant input you hadn't considered and use that information to adjust your resource needs, threats, actions, or contingencies, which is the last step. Or, just do a 5K!

STEP EIGHT: Create a contingency plan.

Make four columns. Label them trigger event, potential additional data needed, action to be taken, and desired outcome. Based on the feedback from your Red Team and the list of threats in your control, make some contingency plans. Remember, Murphy can come calling anytime. What can go wrong probably will, right?

Gotta go snatch that ISIS asshole? Well, you listed "unknown number of enemy on target" as one of the threats. The contingency you label might be that you get on target and discover you're outnumbered. The key indicator, of course, is that you're getting overrun quickly. The action would then be to abort the mission and exfil off the target or call in your quick reaction force of heavily armed, highly motivated killers. And as mentioned, when it makes sense, rehearse for the contingencies.

For example, if I'm preparing for a big keynote or motivational speech, regardless of how many times I've spoken, I'm still highly regimented in my rehearsal process. That includes visualizing not just the win, but what could go wrong. Technology fails. The audience sucks. I suck. Protesters invade the ballroom. The stage collapses. The event is an hour behind schedule, and I have a plane to catch. Who knows? Still gotta have a plan.

Mental Model

The Outcome Pyramid

Here is where we tie it all together. By now you've hopefully identified some areas in your life where you could embrace the suck a bit more. Push the boundaries of your comfort zone. Achieve loftier goals. Be more consistent. Build resilience. Bounce back faster. Get over the shit that doesn't matter. Spend less time and money on pointless crap. Remove the toxic haters standing in your path. Hang out less with Temptation Tiger. Or all of the above.

So now what? Now you've created your Personal Values Manifesto. You know the benefit of living beyond your comfort zone. You're hopefully clearer on your purpose and your why. You've identified clear objectives and you know how to plan like a Navy SEAL. And most important, you know Hell Week sucks. But your purpose, beliefs, and values won't bring you fulfillment unless they drive you to take the necessary actions to achieve your desired results and live your extraordinary life. Let's face it, a person, team, or business has two types of results: *existing outcomes* and *desired outcomes.*

Now let's talk about how to move away from existing results and run passionately toward desired outcomes. The goals that really mean something to you. The things you deeply give a shit about. The stuff that's bigger than you—more significant than your selfish desires that will lead you nowhere.

Let me introduce to you the Embrace the Suck Outcome Pyramid. There are five tiers.

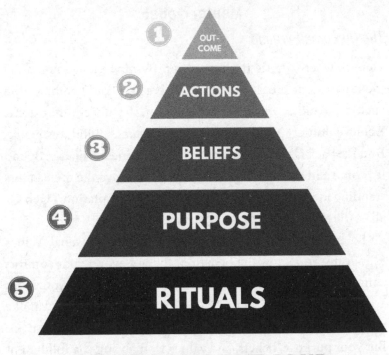

OUTCOME PYRAMID

At the top of the pyramid you have your desired *Outcome*. Again, there are two kinds of outcomes: existing and desired. Maybe that's an overarching life goal of leaving the world a little better that you found it or a shorter-term goal of losing fifteen pounds. Regardless, it must be a clear, concise, quantifiable, and time-bound objective.

The next tier on the pyramid is *Actions*. This is where the planning methodology comes into play. The desired outcome is the result of achieving the objective and the rest of the plan falls into the Actions tier. So, plug that plan into tier two.

The third layer of the pyramid is *Beliefs*. Now we plug in your Personal Values Manifesto. This is where you start asking the questions: Will my beliefs and values drive me to proactively take the actions necessary to achieve my desired outcome. Is that outcome even in line with my beliefs and values? If not, should I even be pursuing it?

The fourth tier is *Purpose*. Your overarching why. Let's say your why is to leave the world a better place than you found it. Ideally, that purpose helps influence your values. Your values fuel you to take the appropriate actions (as part of your plan) to achieve your desired result. Maybe it's starting a nonprofit that helps veterans with PTSD. Boom. The world instantly becomes a better place. Mission accomplished.

The final and most important tier of the pyramid is *Rituals*. For example, let's say your company is going through a major transformation due to a global pandemic—hypothetically speaking, of course. You have several key strategic imperatives associated with this transformation—your desired Outcome. Therefore, the company needs to take new actions, refine procedures, implement a new operating model, and change the culture to achieve winning results. The Actions. In this case, sometimes there is a need for newly defined Beliefs. Not a shift in core values, but rather a new way of thinking—putting away the old and embracing the new. Like leadership and business expert Marshall Goldsmith's game-changing book *What Got You Here Won't Get You There*. Same concept.

You must then ensure that any new beliefs or actions taken align with the company's overall purpose. Finally, you need to ensure that all existing or needed rituals support the purpose, beliefs, and values. So, if your company needs to be more innovative to maintain its competitive advantage, you need people doing cool innovative stuff. If there are no rituals associated with innovation, you need to design them. For example, start an innovation lab during working hours each week where people can work on whatever project they want, as long as those projects are associated with the company's goals and objectives.

The Outcome Pyramid is a model to ensure you are doing the right things for the right reasons to achieve better goals and drive desired outcomes. Not hoping tomorrow will be better, but mandating that it will be so. It's how you model mindset and behavior for violent execution. And remember, a good plan executed violently today is far better than a perfect plan next week. Why? Because there is no such thing as a perfect plan, and, chances are, tomorrow will be different, bringing new challenges and new opportunities.

Great, So What Now?

Use the models! They can be used in any environment from DIY home projects and mastering the art of stilt-walking to building a new business, raising a child, or battling depression or obesity.

Living life beyond your comfort zone sucks even more if you don't have a plan and your values don't align with what you are trying to accomplish. So make sure they do.

Questions to ask yourself:

When a shiny thing passes by or a new idea pops into my head, am I thoughtful in whether to pursue it? Do I create a plan or jump into the abyss?

In my pursuit of personal and professional goals, how often do I ask myself if those goals align with my beliefs and values?

If I have a goal that aligns with my values, do I have the appropriate rituals that support my beliefs in pursuing that goal?

Do I have the right mindset, the tenacity and resilience, and the will to win necessary to accomplish my goals? If not, why the fuck not?

10

WE'RE ALL GOING TO DIE, SO GET OFF YOUR ASS AND EXECUTE

Cowards die many times before their deaths;
The valiant never taste of death but once.

—WILLIAM SHAKESPEARE, *JULIUS CAESAR*

Recent studies show that humans have a 100 percent mortality rate. Taxes are the only other certainty in life. But we fear the unknown of death. The when. The how. The why. Who will be by our side? What will we have accomplished? Is there another life after this one? A heaven? Or is this short life all we get? The answers to these questions all lie in our own unique beliefs. The bottom line is that we have no time to waste.

As Tecumseh said, "Be not like those whose hearts are filled with the fear of death, so they weep, and pray for a little more time to live their lives over again in a different way. Sing your death song and die like a hero going home." To sum up his words: live life so you have little to no regrets when your time card gets punched. Live a life of meaning, of responsibility, of giving to others. Live your life so that you have no reason to fear the end, so when death comes, you can say, "I'm ready."

Death scares us. We have a hard time embracing its reality, so we avoid talking about it, thinking about it, and even acknowledging it when we lose those we love. Yet, in reality, death is the light by which the shadow of all life's meaning is measured. Without death, without an end or a journey over the great divide to something better, life has no significance. As tribal leaders used to say in ancient Afghanistan, *narik ta*. Meaning, what's the point? Without death, everything would seem inconsequential, all experiences arbitrary, all values and metrics would be zero.

As I mentioned, the 9/11 attacks occurred two days before my class began the advanced portion of SEAL training. And as we all know, 9/11 changed everything. Especially for our servicemen and women. That's when we all knew we'd be going to war. For how long, nobody knew. At what cost? We assumed a very high cost, but at the time we couldn't fathom it would be this high.

When you graduate from SEAL training you feel invincible. But you're not. I distinctly remember saying goodbye to my parents the day I deployed to Iraq in 2003. We were the first task unit of 30 SEALs going in-country to hunt the bad guys. My parents were staying at the W Hotel in downtown San Diego. They'd flown in to see me off. Their son was going downrange to take the fight to the enemy. When it was time to say our final goodbyes, my mom turned to me and placed her hands gently on both sides of my face. She couldn't speak, but her body language said enough. Tears streamed down her face as she smiled a smile of fear and pain, chin quivering. She was saying goodbye. Not good-bye like, "I'll see you in six months." But "Goodbye."

Despite what you see in the movies, SEALs aren't immortal. We are very, very mortal. And I hate to break it to you, but we don't breathe fire or eat glass either. And those of us still standing feel guilty every day for being alive when our brothers aren't. But if you could ask the fallen if they had any regrets, they'd say not one. They sang their death songs and died like heroes going home.

As King Richard I said in an address to his men during the Third Crusade in 1192:

> Our destiny awaits us, but even though we are outnumbered do not fear the hand of death. Everybody dies eventually. Not everyone can choose to end their time with glory and honor. To stand as brothers in arms, shoulder-to-shoulder, shield-by-shield, sword upon sword, battling our enemies for freedom and the greater good. That my friends is a glory worth fighting for. That my brothers is an honor worth dying for.

San Diego, California
June 2005

I yawned as I poured a cup of coffee. I grabbed the remote and turned on the TV, tuning in to CNN or Fox News, I can't remember. And there they were: Mike, Axe, and Danny in images that had been recovered from Taliban propaganda websites. They were SEAL warriors who'd made the ultimate sacrifice on the battlefield. The coffee mug slipped from my hand and shattered on the floor. Tears welled in my eyes as I watched the report. Two weeks later, I attended Mike's funeral at Calverton National Cemetery in Suffolk County, New York.

The day began at the funeral parlor where attendees came to pay their respects. It was pouring rain. When we exited the funeral parlor, six of Mike's teammates carried his coffin to the hearse. Local Long Island police and NYC firefighters were standing in ranks, saluting at full attention in the rain. It was overwhelming. A procession of dozens of cars proceeded to the church. The highways were shut down and lined with fire trucks for miles. They were in pairs, one on each side of the road, ladders raised suspending the largest American flags I've ever seen. After the ceremony at the church, the procession headed to the National Cemetery.

Michael Murphy and I had been in BUD/S class 235 together until he was rolled to 236 for stress fractures. His was my second Navy funeral and first SEAL funeral, and it was the most powerful yet gut wrenching thing to witness. Folded flags were presented to his mother, Maureen, and his fiancée, Heather. One of his teammates kneeled humbly in front of Maureen, head bowed, arms extended, holding the flag high. He didn't move or look up until she accepted the flag, torn but stoic. His platoon then lined up, each man walking up to the casket to say farewell. They each pulled their Trident pins from their chests and slammed them into the wood of the casket; the gold pins lining the smooth mahogany lid symbolized their brotherhood. Each teammate, friend, and family member lost a piece of themselves in that moment.

Operation Red Wings was a counterinsurgent mission in Kunar province in Afghanistan that involved four Navy SEALs. Murphy and two other SEALs, Danny Dietz and Matthew Axelson, were killed in the fighting, in addition to sixteen US special operations soldiers (eight SEALs and eight 160th Army Special

Operations Aviations) who were killed when their helicopter was shot down while attempting to extract the SEALs. At the time, it was both the largest loss of life for US forces since the invasion began and the largest loss for the SEALs since the Vietnam War. Marcus Luttrell was the only surviving SEAL. He fought his way to a local village where he was protected. Eventually, villagers sent an emissary to the closest military base, which allowed a rescue team to locate him. The story is captured in his riveting book, *Lone Survivor*, which became a 2013 blockbuster movie of the same name.

Mike was the commander of a four-man reconnaissance team. They were on a mission to kill or capture a top Taliban leader, Ahmad Shah, who led a group of insurgents known as the "Mountain Tigers." The team was dropped off by helicopter in a remote, mountainous area east of Asadabad in Kunar, near the Pakistan border. After an initially successful infiltration, local goat herders stumbled upon the SEALs' hiding place. Unable to verify any hostile intent from the herders, the team cut them loose. Hostile locals, possibly the goat herders they released, alerted nearby Taliban forces, who soon surrounded and attacked the team from an elevated position. A raging gunfight ensued. After Mike radioed for help, an MH-47 Chinook helicopter loaded with reinforcements was dispatched to rescue the team, but was shot down with an RPG, killing all sixteen personnel aboard.

Mike was killed after he left his cover position and went to a clearing away from the mountains—exposing himself to a hail of gunfire—to get a clear signal to contact headquarters and relay the dire situation and request immediate support for his team. He dropped the satellite phone after being shot multiple times, but picked it up and finished the call. While being shot, he signed off saying, "Thank You," then continued fighting from his exposed position until he died from his wounds.

Mike, Danny, and Axe fought like warrior poets and were killed in action, taking more than half of the large Taliban force with them. Marcus Luttrell was the only US survivor. Mike was awarded the Medal of Honor for his heroism and selflessness on the mountain that day. All three of Mike's men were awarded the Navy's second highest honor, the Navy Cross, for their part in the battle, making theirs the most decorated Navy SEAL Team in history at the time.

Mike's eulogy was a powerful testament to who he was as a son, a warrior, a teammate, and a man.

One Mile off the East Coast of Africa
4:30 A.M.

The large dhow listed back and forth violently as the sea raged beneath us. I was huddled under a large plastic tarp on the aft upper deck of the boat with my teammates Scotty and Jeff and our interpreter. It was pouring rain and we were soaking wet. I can't divulge the purpose of our mission, but we'd been living on this piece of crap for about a week now, eating homemade pancakes and drinking sweet tea. Our toilet was a hole in the back deck that opened out to the crystal blue water. By now my limited Swahili was actually passable. We wore only shorts and T-shirts. Also in our possession were two large black Pelican cases full of weapons and sat comm radios. Our vessel was staffed with a relatively capable ragtag crew of nine locals. The sea state seemed to be getting worse and we were contemplating calling for extraction from the Special Warfare Combatant-Craft Crewmen (SWCC) team on standby many miles south of our location.

"Man, we're really embracing the suck now, huh brother?" I said to Scotty. He was next to me under the tarp, our only protection from the downpour. My knees and elbows were raw and bloody from sliding around on the dirty deck as the dhow swayed back and forth. Infection imminent!

"Do you guys smell smoke?" Jeff asked. "Oh shit, yeah I do," I responded. We threw off the tarp and moved over to the ladder that went down to the second deck and then to the engine room below. Through the opening, we could see flames shooting out of the engine room. "Hey guys, check this out," I said.

"Ummm, well that's no good," Jeff said with his usual mischievous grin (but with a slight bit of concern quickly developing in his facial expression). Four of our crew began bucketing water into the engine room. Another guy was then tossing the water back out. This was quickly becoming a goat rope. A total shitshow.

"Geezuz . . . let's get down there and help these guys," Scotty said with an eye roll. We headed down while Jeff got on the radio to our SWCC team. He ended the call by saying, "If you see three white guys floating in shark-infested waters clinging to wooden pallets, that's us." Luckily, we put out the fire and the sea state eventually calmed. We felt like true sailors once again.

Both Scotty and Jeff have gone over the great divide, now residing in Valhalla. Many years after our Africa trip, Scotty was among the four brave Americans killed in the cowardly suicide bombing attack in Syria on January 16, 2019. Several years prior, Jeff was found dead on the floor of his apartment. Cause of death was unknown. I look forward to the day we'll all reunite and tell tall tales of life in the Teams.

In 2012, I was a cast member on Mark Burnett and Dick Wolf's CBS reality series *Stars Earn Stripes*. The basic premise of the TV show was to pair celebrities such as Nick Lachey, Dean Cain, Terry Crews, Laila Ali, Todd Palin, and Picabo Street with former special operators to compete in missions. My friend and teammate Chris Kyle was the other SEAL on the show. Soon after the show aired—on February 2, 2013—Chris and his friend Chad Littlefield were murdered. Chris and Chad were shot and killed while walking downrange to set up targets at a gun range near Chalk Mountain, Texas. Eddie Ray Routh, a twenty-five-year-old Marine whom Chris was mentoring due to PTSD, killed them both. The case attracted national attention due to Kyle's fame as author of the best-selling autobiography *American Sniper*, published in 2012. Clint Eastwood later directed a film adaptation based on Kyle's book. Taya Kyle, Chris's widow and mother of their two children, carries on the name as a best-selling author and veteran advocate. And, yes, she's a total badass.

Death comes for us all. For the most part, we don't know exactly when. Why waste a precious moment on pointless activities and relationships that leave us hollow and unfulfilled? Why leave our list of regrets to chance? Why not spend more time giving to causes greater than ourselves? Why not take total ownership and plan our extraordinary life with the end in mind?

Mental Model

Working Backward from the End

The second habit Stephen Covey covers in his groundbreaking book *The 7 Habits of Highly Effective People* is "Begin With the End in Mind." Close your eyes and think about someone giving your eulogy. Do they talk about how much money you made? Your job titles? How big your house was? How many cars you owned? That you kicked major ass at *Fortnite*? That you made Dean's Roll every semester? That you not once, not twice, but three times had a clever tweet go viral? That you had thousands of Instagram followers?

If you're like most decent human beings, that's probably not what you're envisioning. You're probably imagining them talking about your *virtues*. You likely imagine a trusted friend talking about your character and relationships. The kind of husband, father, wife, mother, and friend you were. How hard you worked to give your kids not only a good life, but a sense of purpose and a sound moral compass. How you still did little romantic gestures for your spouse, even though you'd been hitched for decades. How you'd give the shirt off your back to your buddies. You probably imagine him sharing stories both funny and sad that highlight your integrity, kindness, and curiosity and the effect you had on the lives of others.

According to Covey, before you can live a good, meaningful life, you've got to know what that looks like. When we know how we want people to talk about us at the end of our life, we can start taking action now to make that scenario a reality later. With the end in mind, we know what we need to do day-to-day and week-to-week to get there. We know how to execute our mission plan.

Now it's time to make your Embrace the Suck Regrets Checklist. Use the model below to ensure you live an extraordinary life with no regrets that is full of purpose, giving more of yourself to others, and leaves a legacy that makes the world a better place. I've provided some themes, but I leave it to you to customize this for yourself.

WHEN IT COMES TO . . .	I NEVER WANT TO REGRET . . .
Family	
Personal relationships	
Health	
Professional career	
Giving back	
Taking calculated risk	
My values	
My purpose	
Being bold	
Loving fiercely	

You can take it from here.

Great, So What Now?

The point is, we're all going to have to sing our death song someday. What will the words of your song be? What mark do you want to leave on the world? What do you absolutely not want to regret on the day you pass? Will you reflect back and realize you didn't take many risks and stayed safely in your village? Or will you know that you left everything you had on the battlefield of life?

The choice is yours.

Questions to ask yourself:

Am I willing to purposefully suffer to seek true fulfillment and happiness?

In my current state, what would people truly say about me after I'm gone?

What am I willing to change about myself to live by my eulogy virtues?

Do I prioritize the stuff that aligns with my values and the values of those I love?

What do I not want to regret when this life comes to an end?

EPILOGUE

TRANSFORM YOUR MIND, LIVE EXTRAORDINARILY

Let everything happen to you. Beauty and terror. Just keep going. No feeling is final.

—RAINER MARIA RILKE

Now, my friend, it's time for you to step forth onto your battlefield and take the fight to the enemy. To go to war with yourself. Time to build resilience muscles, set and achieve lofty goals, pursue excellence and innovation in all you do, and master the art of maximum performance. I'd like to leave you with a few Navy SEAL sayings (some you now know) to keep you focused and energized. You can use them as fuel for your journey. Embrace them. Share them with others. Do what you must each day to embrace the suck and live an extraordinary life. Through discipline and resilience, you'll win this battle and many more to come.

Good luck!

Fail-Safe Principles to Transform Your Mind and Live an Extraordinary Life

Embrace the suck. Accept life's challenges for what they are—opportunities for growth and development. Make the choice to lean in, not run away.

The only easy day was yesterday. There are no easy days for high-performing individuals or teams pursuing an existence of excellence. Tackle challenges head on, controlling what you can and ignoring what you can't.

Get comfortable being uncomfortable. Push the boundaries and confines of your comfort zone every chance you get. The more you do, the more your comfort zone expands.

Persevere and thrive on adversity. When you face adversity, just walk right up and give it a big old bear hug. Befriend it. Recertify yourself as a savage every chance you get.

It pays to be a winner. We all have a different definition of what winning means to us. Clearly define your objectives, have a plan, and dominate your battlefield.

In the absence of orders, I will take charge. Don't wait for someone else to dictate your life for you. Take charge. Discipline and accountability are the true path to enlightenment and fulfillment.

Stay in your three-foot world. Focus on what is in your immediate control and deprioritize everything else. This allows you to prioritize and execute where you have the maximum impact.

Demand discipline. Expect innovation. Disciplined and creative people achieve more of their goals. Don't waste time on things that don't align with your values and desired outcomes.

Slow is smooth and smooth is fast. Improving performance in any aspect of life takes time. Get the little things right first, then keep moving the goalposts.

Eat the elephant one bite at a time. When it comes to achieving big goals and navigating life's obstacles, when we have too many priorities, we have no priorities. Prioritize and execute.

Uncompromising integrity is my standard. Integrity and trust have a direct and measurable impact on personal performance and the success of any team or relationship.

Never out of the fight. I believe in this life philosophy so much that I have it tattooed on my arm in Latin. *Numquam Proelia Derelinquam.* It needs no interpretation.

ACKNOWLEDGMENTS

Where do I begin? I learned the first time around that writing a book is a complex journey involving many people—it's a team effort in every sense of the word. The timing of this book's release lands at the conclusion of a very challenging year for people across the globe. Challenges that will have ripple effects for years to come. But my inspiration began with the humbling experience of being blessed with the opportunity to serve alongside some of the greatest warriors that the world has ever known. Our servicemen and servicewomen—and their families—who give so much to a cause greater than themselves, will always touch me with great emotion. They stand ready to answer our nation's call and defend us against enemies who wish to destroy us. And some, of course, give their lives. We sleep peacefully at night because of the brave men and women who willingly run to the sound of gunfire and set aside their own selfish desires to protect our way of life and the freedoms we enjoy.

I could never have accomplished this rewarding effort without the loving support of my amazing wife, Nicole. She is my best friend, business partner, and commanding officer. Thank you to my three amazing children, Tyler, Parker Rose, and Ryder— and, of course, to our new bundle of joy due in January 2021.

We will soon have a full fire team! Writing is a creative process that often requires quiet and solitude, not something that comes easily in a full household of five amidst a global pandemic. Without the uncompromising support and leadership of my wife, the completion of this project may not have come to fruition.

I owe special thanks to my amazing team. My literary agent, Farley Chase, who took a chance on me once again. His guidance, feedback, and advice continue to prove invaluable as I refine my craft as an author. Thank you to my editor, Dan Ambrosio, and the unbelievably talented team at Hachette Book Group.

And last but not least, a sincere thank you to my Navy SEAL brothers who participated in this project. To David Goggins, who was generous enough to contribute the foreword. David continues to inspire people all over the world—I'm proud to call him BUD/S classmate, Team Five teammate, and friend. Special thanks to my warrior brother Jason Redman for allowing me to tell his riveting story of survival, perseverance, and resilience. Your books have inspired many to reform their ideas about resilience and overcoming adversity. Looking forward to our new adventures. Thank you to Mark Owen (badass pipe hitter, former teammate, and number one *New York Times* best-selling author of *No Easy Day* and *No Hero*) for your friendship and guidance over the past twenty years.

Everyone who contributed to this effort further solidifies the fact that nothing of any great value can be accomplished by any one individual. It takes a team.

RESOURCES

Baumeister, Roy F., and John Tierney. *Willpower: Rediscovering the Greatest Human Strength*. New York: Penguin Books, 2001.

Clear, James. "Let Your Values Drive Your Choices." Accessed April 23, 2020. https://jamesclear.com/values-choices.

Covington, Martin. "Self-Worth Theory: Retrospection and Prospects." In *Handbook of Motivation at School*, edited by Kathryn R. Wentzel and Allan Wigfield. New York: Routledge, 2009.

Crum, Alia, and Thomas Crum. "Stress Can Be a Good Thing If You Know How to Use It." *Harvard Business Review*, September 3, 2015. https://hbr.org/2015/09/stress-can-be-a-good-thing-if-you-know-how-to-use-it.

Dweck, Carol S. *Mindset: The New Psychology of Success*. New York: Ballantine Books, 2006.

Gleeson, Brent. *TakingPoint: A Navy SEAL's 10 Fail-Safe Principles for Leading Through Change*. New York: Touchstone, 2018.

Goggins, David. *Can't Hurt Me: Master Your Mind and Defy the Odds*. Austin, Texas: Lioncrest, 2018.

Goldsmith, Marshall, with Mark Reiter. *What Got You Here Won't Get You There: How Successful People Become Even More Successful*. New York: Hachette, 2007.

Hillenbrand, Laura. *Unbroken: A World War II Story of Survival, Resilience, and Redemption.* New York: Random House, 2010.

Honnold, Alex, with David Roberts. *Alone on the Wall.* New York: Norton, 2016.

Konnikova, Maria. "How People Learn to Become Resilient." *New Yorker*, February 11, 2016. https://www.newyorker.com/science/maria-konnikova/the-secret-formula-for-resilience.

Mangurian, Glenn E. "Realizing What You're Made Of." *Harvard Business Review*, March 2007. https://hbr.org/2007/03/realizing-what-youre-made-of.

Owen, Mark. *No Easy Day: The Firsthand Account of the Mission That Killed Osama Bin Laden.* New York: Penguin Books, 2012.

ABOUT THE AUTHOR

BRENT GLEESON is a Navy SEAL combat veteran and successful businessman. Upon leaving SEAL Team Five, Brent turned his discipline and battlefield lessons to the world of business and has become an award-winning entrepreneur, best-selling author, and acclaimed speaker and consultant on topics including leadership, building high-performance teams, culture, resilience, and organizational transformation.

Brent is the founder and CEO of TakingPoint Leadership, a progressive leadership and organizational development consulting firm with a focus on business transformation and building high-performance cultures. Brent was named a top ten CEO by *Entrepreneur* magazine in 2013.

Brent is a respected thought leader in leadership and organizational transformation. His expertise is both real-world and academic in nature, having built several high-growth organizations.

Brent holds degrees in finance and economics from Southern Methodist University, certificates in English and history from the University of Oxford in England, and a graduate business degree from the University of San Diego.

He is the author of *TakingPoint: A Navy SEAL's 10 Fail-Safe Principles for Leading Through Change*, which was a number one new release on Amazon in organizational change and business structural adjustment.